Fascist Yoga

'Anything Stewart Home writes, thinks, fancies, or loathes intrigues me. Reading Home is a special experience, dizzying. Home turns things upside down and shakes them up, and sometimes he recites his work standing on his head. Engaging with him, you might land on your head, also.'

—Lynne Tillman, author of *Weird Fucks* and *Mothercare*

'With this scabrous broadside, Stewart Home exposes Hatha yoga's political shadow. His painstaking research reveals a hidden, decidedly inauthentic history as murky as it is intriguing. Teasing a thread from a pair of dhoti pants, soon the whole garment threatens to fall apart before our eyes.'

—Matthew Ingram, author of *The Garden* and *Retreat*

'The author's desire to stand on his head led to this book, but there is nothing upside down about his exposure of the plastic gurus and spiritual sex pests to be found in these pages. Intense, funny, always original – there is nobody quite like the brilliant Stewart Home.'

—John King, author of *The Football Factory* and *Human Punk*

'With an energy and style that only he could muster, Stewart Home eviscerates the two dominant manias of our era – individual self-optimisation and collective neo-fascism – and, reading their entrails, finds they share a common ancestor.'

—Tom McCarthy, author of *Remainder* and *The Making of Incarnation*

Fascist Yoga

Grifters, Occultists,
White Supremacists and
the New Order in Wellness

Stewart Home

First published 2025 by Pluto Press
New Wing, Somerset House, Strand, London WC2R 1LA
and Pluto Press, Inc.
1930 Village Center Circle, 3-834, Las Vegas, NV 89134

www.plutobooks.com

Copyright © Stewart Home 2025

The right of Stewart Home to be identified as the author of this work has been asserted in accordance with the Copyright, Designs and Patents Act 1988.

British Library Cataloguing in Publication Data
A catalogue record for this book is available from the British Library

ISBN 978 0 7453 5112 4 Paperback
ISBN 978 0 7453 5118 6 PDF
ISBN 978 0 7453 5113 1 EPUB

This book is printed on paper suitable for recycling and made from fully managed and sustained forest sources. Logging, pulping and manufacturing processes are expected to conform to the environmental standards of the country of origin.

Typeset by Stanford DTP Services, Northampton, England

Simultaneously printed in the United Kingdom and United States of America

EU GPSR Authorised Representative
LOGOS EUROPE, 9 rue Nicolas Poussin, 17000, LA ROCHELLE, France
Email: Contact@logoseurope.eu

Contents

Introduction   1

PART I   HAPPY BABY: A GRUBBY GURU TAKES US ALL TO THE CLEANERS

1   Did Pierre Bernard Invent Yoga in California at the Start of the Twentieth Century?   17
2   The Great Oom and White Power   25

PART II   WARRIOR ONE, TWO AND THREE: FASCISM + YOGA = FASCIST YOGA (THE 1920s TO THE 1940s)

3   Guido Keller and the Rijeka Yoga Group   38
4   Military Theorist Major J. F. C. Fuller, Whose Concept of Blitzkrieg Became Standard Practice in Nazi Warfare   47
5   Bengal Lancer and Hitler Aficionado Francis Yeats-Brown   54
6   Jakob Wilhelm Hauer and His Influence on the Architect of the Nazi Holocaust Heinrich Himmler   66
7   Mircea Eliade, Julius Evola, Savitri Devi – National Socialism as a Religion and the Yoga of Power   72

PART III   DOWNWARD DOG: OCCULT MADNESS AND YOGIC TELEVANGELISM (MODERN POSTURAL PRACTICE IN THE POST-WAR ERA)

8   Paul Dukes, Francis Yeats-Brown (Again) and Theos Bernard, Spreading the Great Oom's Gospel in the Post-war Years   90

9	Indra Devi and Her Editors at Prentice Hall	96
10	Harvey Day, a Hack Who Found Success with Books on Yoga	104
11	Desmond Dunne aka Occultist James Lee-Richardson and His Mail Order Yoga Course	116
12	Richard Hittleman and Yogic Televangelism	129
13	Pull the Wool Over Your Own Eyes with Frank Rudolph Young, the 'Einstein' of Occult Yoga	138

Conclusion 153

Notes 157
Bibliography 186
Index 201

Introduction

While the Covid pandemic may, to a degree, have offered a gateway for yoga's repressed fascist past to resurface in the form of anti-vax and anti-masking politicking, leading in turn to the explosion of QAnon and other far-right conspiracy theories, the signs of where things were headed could already be seen. In fact, in my experience, fascism and fascists can pop up in the most unexpected places – and not just in yoga. Shortly after the turn of the millennium, I was researching my dead mother's life. I tracked down a man she'd known called Bill Hopkins, who I understood to have been a successful antiques dealer in London's Portobello Road.

Over generous shots of Talisker whiskey, Hopkins told me he'd met my mother in the early sixties at Murray's Cabaret Club, where she worked as showgirl and hostess. The conversation was animated, drifting off in odd directions as the evening wore on. By the time Hopkins observed Hitler was the most influential figure of the twentieth century, it had dawned on me that he was a fascist. Years later, I learned Hopkins was not just any old fascist, but one who in his political heyday had been plugged into an international far-right terrorist network that used a bombing campaign to wreak havoc during Italy's Years of Lead.[1]

My mother had been a beatnik and then a hippie. I knew many of her friends and they were generally apolitical. Some had worked for Hopkins doing house clearances and, when quizzed, were insistent they were unaware of his far-right views. In a way, my experience with Hopkins was repeated when I started gym yoga classes, although it took me a lot longer to understand that at least some of the roots of modern postural practice are to be found in white supremacy and fascist ideology.

One of the things my mother's hippie set and many of those engaged with yoga share (or shared) with fascists like Bill Hopkins is a worldview grounded in essentialism and anti-empiricism. Many fascists, hippies and yogis act and speak as if there is a natural essence to everything that trumps science-based evidence. In short, what they believe to be true is – at least as far as they were concerned – not only true but irrefutable. Likewise, fascists, hippies and modern yoga all owe a debt to the work of occultist Helena Blavatsky (1831–91), regardless of whether they are fully conversant with her ideas about 'root races'.

Quite a number of things happened before I began to think about the relationship between modern postural practice and the far right. I'll run through some of that before moving on to the serious business of fascist yoga, starting with a few personal experiences.

Yoga classes were offered as part of the gym membership I had back in the day and because I wanted to learn to stand on my head I started attending them. Like many others of my generation, I'd first come across yoga as a child, having seen it on a TV programme hosted by an American named Richard Hittleman. If I was bored, I'd sometimes try the exercises that Hittleman – who seemed more of a salesman than a mystic – had women in leotards demonstrate on his *Yoga For Health* programme.

Postural practice was not my principal exercise interest but it was the closest thing to gymnastics tuition included in my gym membership. The sports club was a few minutes walk from my flat, and going there provided a good break from spending the day at home working on a computer. It was one of the gym's yoga instructors, Jen, who first got me thinking about yoga as a cult activity when, in 2012, she broke with the Anusara practice that had been the basis of her teaching.

Anusara is a style of yoga invented in America by John Friend. In 2012, a scandal blew up around him, with accusations made that he had pursued affairs with his students and employees. Although Friend – unlike some other yogis – doesn't appear to have forced himself on those who said no to his sexual advances, there were clearly consent issues around his behaviour. Friend also had his employees receive packages of illegal drugs on his behalf, and played fast and loose with their pension contributions, ascribing the latter to a 'clerical error'.[2] Friend was also exposed as the head of an otherwise all-female Wiccan coven that performed nude rituals.

Had I seen a copy of Friend's *Anusara Yoga Teacher Training Manual* before going to my first postural class, it would have probably put me off attending.[3] At the end of the Introduction, Friend states: 'throughout the *Manual* I have arbitrarily referred to God, the Absolute in the masculine and God, the relative or individual being of consciousness (in the form of the student) in the feminine.' Later, the book turns to 'Health Concerns'. Here, Friend recommends inversions, alongside hip-openers, for constipation. If the student is flexible enough, they can engage in a sitting-forward bend to rectify a detached retina. As should be obvious, Friend's advice is based on fables: there is no scientific evidence that a single yoga pose can help cure a specific – and often complex – medical condition. Indeed, the various 'scientific' studies of yoga that conclude it provides health benefits merely demonstrate that exercise is good for you, rather than proving yoga is a superior form of exercise. What yoga can do to improve your health hasn't really been tested because there is no agreement about what yoga actually is.

In the years following the storm around Friend, a succession of yoga scandals broke. How they impacted on individual teachers varied according to their relationship to the latest guru who'd been exposed as having feet of clay. Since there was no hot yoga at my gym, the instructors there didn't have much of a connection to Bikram Choudhury, a narcissistic clown who between 2014 and 2020 gained notoriety due to a series of sexual assault cases brought against him. More recently, avowed feminist Katie Griggs – aka Guru Jagat – gained the limelight by leaping to the defence of sexual predator Harbhajan Singh Khalsa, a one-time customs official who in the 1960s created the kundalini style of yoga taught by Griggs. Griggs, who died of a heart attack in 2021 at the age of 41, was also exposed as exploiting her employees and engaging in Covid denial and anti-masking conspiracies.[4]

Recent high-profile abuses of power such as these, however, only scratch the surface in terms of the fragile – indeed, imaginary – foundations on which modern yoga is based. The more I learned about modern yoga, the more I came to view it as an invented tradition with parallels to Wicca and witchcraft, which are also recent concoctions.[5] More generally, recent years have seen a growing interest in various invented traditions, many of which are tied to forms of nationalism, with yoga becoming entwined with its Indian variant. That said, yoga as practised in the Western world appears to me to be a thoroughly occidental pursuit.

Initially, I was mildly surprised by the extent to which some of those teaching me modern postural practice banged on about their discipline being an ancient Indian tradition. According to them, the practice originated on the Indian subcontinent and is therefore Indian. That is not how I see it, but this disjunction of perspective arises in part from how one defines and understands the term 'yoga' – I would argue the use of the word in English should not be confused with its many meanings in Sanskrit.[6] Moreover, it is worth stressing again that there is no agreement on what modern postural yoga is, and that many different exercise systems are practised under its rubric.

My impetus for looking specifically at the links between yoga and fascism was a 2016 article by Sanjiv Bhattacharya entitled 'Call Me A Racist, But Don't Say I'm A Buddhist'.[7] At the top was a picture of a man named only as Eric – later identified as Eric Lyle Atwood[8] – in a half-lotus pose, his hands in a meditation *mudra* shape with a neo-fascist Celtic cross flag behind him and a 'Make America Great Again' cap resting on his right knee.

Bhattacharya was profiling Atwood and other members of the American Freedom Party, who saw getting Donald Trump elected as the first step towards creating a white American ethnostate. Atwood became the star of the piece, eclipsing his political boss William Johnson. From Bhattacharya's perspective, Atwood's story seemed counterintuitive: 'Eric isn't your average Nazi. He trained as a spiritualist. He has taught meditation. He brought his tarot cards in case I wanted a reading ... Eric still meditates and practises yoga.'

To me, this description sounded disturbingly like your average countercultural fascist. For decades, I'd been aware of musicians whose fanbases consisted largely of rune-loving, tarot card-reading, spiritualist-inclined, Hitler-obsessed, racist reactionaries. This pool of countercultural fascists is often associated with the underground neofolk scene. Over the years, some of the musicians involved have been accused of being neo-Nazis, although they consistently deny this. Nevertheless, Spencer Sunshine's recent book *Neo-Nazi Terrorism and Countercultural Fascism* meticulously documents the decades-long links cultivated by two such musicians – Boyd Rice and Michael Moynihan – to the violent American far right.[9]

Ringing further alarm bells for me was Atwood's stated desire to make it big with a rock band he was forming called

The Beach Goys. Since I already knew odd parts of the underground rock scene were riddled with neo-Nazis, it struck me as possible that the yoga world was similarly afflicted. The same source that provided Atwood's surname also noted his involvement with the Rise Above Movement (RAM), a southern Californian white supremacist group that has played a key role in promoting 'active clubs' across North America. Active clubs are organisations set up to enable white supremacists to practice mixed martial arts and develop their 'warrior spirit'.[10] Atwood and others around him were therefore in a prime position to inject yoga into the North American active-club scene — although whether this actually happened still isn't known to me.

I was already concerned by several aspects of the yoga world: the cult-like devotion it inspires, repeated sexual abuse by teachers, the jockeying between multiple governing bodies for power, and the occult-saturated health misinformation spewed forth by some of those who taught modern postural practice at my local gym. After reading Bhattacharya's article, I realised that fascist connections could in all likelihood be added to the list of things that worried me about modern yoga. I therefore took a dive into yoga literature and, a few months later, in January 2017, began blogging about subjects related to this.

Historical essays relating to fascist yoga got more reaction than anything else I posted at the time. That said, there was less interest in material about the Rashtriya Swayamsevak Sangh — a precursor to India's current Bharatiya Janata Party (BJP) government — whose leaders proclaimed their admiration and support for Hitler when he was in power, than reportage of European fascist yogis. In terms of yoga's occult strands, my coverage was mostly contemporary. Having blogged on these subjects for two years, I eventually decided I should reorganise some of the material I'd posted into a book. Before doing so, though, I needed to do further research into the historical entanglements of yoga and occultism.

Some may consider my timing poor. Less than 18 months after I knocked my blogging about modern yoga on the head, the *Conspirituality* podcast started up and quickly achieved considerable acclaim, including for addressing far-right influences on the yoga world. Eventually, the makers of the podcast went on to write the book *Conspirituality: How New Age Conspiracy Theories Became A Health Threat*.[11] The podcast and book had a tangible influence on mainstream media coverage of yogis and other new age figures jumping aboard the anti-vax, anti-masking, far-right bandwagon.

That said, while those behind the podcast clearly wanted to save modern postural practice from the far right – on many levels, a worthy project – my critique was broader and more likely to provoke anger in yoga circles, fascist or not. Despite initially hoping to separate modern postural practice from the pseudo-science and grooming likely to lead people down conspiracy rabbit holes, I gradually came to understand that sorting the postural wheat from the chaff was a tall order. The combination of essentialism and anti-empiricism that is prevalent among modern yoga practitioners makes them particularly susceptible to both occult delusions and fascist conspiritorialism. Over time, this has led me to the position that it is more practical to simply take up an alternative exercise regime than attempt to sanitise modern postural practice.

I find it depressing that many yoga instructors present discredited medieval ideas about 'bodily energy centres' and 'grids' as some kind of Eastern scientific accomplishment, while ignoring the fact that the Indian subcontinent is today a hotbed of technological achievement. What is talked up as 'Eastern' wisdom by many modern postural practice teachers is on a par with claiming that alchemy represents the height of occidental science.

In his book *Practice And All Is Coming*, Matthew Remski – the most prominent of the Conspirituality podcast team – addresses sexual abuse and injury with regard to ashtanga yoga specifically. From my point of view, what he says applies to much of modern postural practice. For example:

> Whether loosely or tightly-bounded, temporary or long-lived, every high-demand group thrives on deception. The high-demand group can be deceptive about what its intentions are, and what its leader and core followers are doing. It can be deceptive about the origins of its teaching content. It can be deceptive about money, and the benefits of its programs. It can be deceptive about its history.[12]

In my experience, the overwhelming majority of yoga instructors peddle false historical accounts of what they teach, even if most of them actually appear to believe the drivel they spout. It is partly due to this, along with the fact that the overly subjective, inward-looking mindset fostered by this form of embodied spirituality makes practitioners vulnerable to backward ideologies and cult exploitation, that I regard postural practice as it exists today as having a negative impact on the world.

Given that he is absolutely central to the QAnon conspiracy theory that forms a key part of the story Remski and his team tell, it is unsurprising that recently re-elected American president Donald Trump features prominently in their book *Conspirituality*. While it is extraordinary that Trump is perceived as someone who will 'save' humanity among certain new age circles, historian Christopher H. Evans' linking of 'New Thought' to his brand of right-wing populism is more germane to understanding why the 'Make America Great Again' movement appeals to so many on today's US yoga scene:

The term 'New Thought' signified that one's thoughts could unlock secrets to living a better life ... its belief that individuals possessed a God-given facility to change their life through positive thinking became embedded in mainstream Christianity ... The fusion between New Thought and Christian libertarianism is epitomized by Norman Vincent Peale ... President Donald Trump frequently cites Peale as his major religious influence.[13]

Modern postural practice emerged in part from New Thought, with some figures who loom large in the former's early history – especially William Walker Atkinson, aka Yogi Ramacharaka – having a hand in shaping both. In many ways, moving away from the North American heartland of modern postural practice makes it easier to see some of the influences – other than QAnon and Trump – shaping the ideology of contemporary right-wing yoga practitioners. An illustrative example in this regard is Marco Mandrino, who runs the Hari-Om Yoga School – a Yoga Alliance-affiliated teacher-training business – based in Sezzadio, Italy.

Mandrino, a persistent if not particularly well-known blogger and author, promotes his yoga school as international, with his site providing pages in both Italian and English. While the English-language translations often leave much to be desired in terms of elegant phrasing, what is being said is comprehensible enough. As the blog makes clear, the measures taken to deal with the Covid pandemic didn't go down well with Mandrino: 'Being "Covid Free" means having your mind cleared of reflected clouds of a year and six months of media terrorism and public-health regime ... Hari-Om is authentically Covid Free in the sense that this terrorism has not affected us, we have never backed down.'[14] In a later post, he asserts that 'everything that had a spiritual meaning in Yoga was crushed by anti-pandemic laws.'[15] Tumbling further down the rabbit hole, Mandrino launches into full-fronted attacks on science, such as: 'these priests in white overcoats, just like the medieval inquisitors, would like to silence, imprison and prosecute anyone who does not see reality with their own eyes ... The blaring propaganda of the "Church/Science" has convinced atrophied minds.'[16]

In some posts, Mandrino refers to cultural-cum-political writers. Perhaps unsurprisingly, many of these are heroes of the far right, with Mandrino proclaiming, for example, that 'Gabriele D'Annunzio is one of the personalities of Italian culture who I admire the most.'[17] In light of his admiration for figures such as D'Annunzio, Mandrino's views on 'woke' culture are somewhat predictable:

> The current culture, dominated by the 'woke', is by far the most intolerant ever ... Those who authentically appreciate both cultural and racial differences are aware that we are not all the same (the fact that we are not all equal is not an opinion but a natural truth) ... The new and modern censors have as their myth a horribly 'equal' society where all differences are flattened in favor of a gray mixture without color or differences of gender or race.[18]

Such views chime with those of the far-right *Nouvelle Droite* movement in France (formed in the late 1960s) and the *Terza Posizione* in Italy (late 1970s), which is to be expected given that they shared Mandrino's interest in the likes of fascist-friendly writers such as René Guénon and Julius Evola (who we will meet in Chapter 7). More recently, the far-right Italian social movement CasaPound, which briefly turned itself into a political party, has operated in the same ideological waters. Most of those involved in such scenes would deny they are fascists, and it is unnecessary to apply this term to them in order to stand in opposition to their reactionary politics and faux-elitist contempt for the rest of humanity – something that is clearly evident in Mandrino's assertion in his writing that the 'dormant masses' are 'guinea pigs' and 'zombies'.

The reason Mandrino merits inclusion here is precisely because he is not high-profile in the yoga world, but rather typical of it. As a small businessman with a yoga school that churns out teachers, he can be seen as an everyday example of yoga entrepreneurship. The two weeks' training required for certification as a teacher with Mandrino costs €1,600 (as of 2024), on top of which students pay for on-site food and accommodation. In other words, anyone with around $2,500 and two weeks to spare can become a certified yoga teacher, having also imbibed at least some of their instructor's anti-scientific, right-wing worldview.

While Mandrino may have self-consciously introduced elements of European traditionalist ideology into his yoga practice, he is still very much a product of yoga's evolution from the carnival-style ballyhoo of Pierre Bernard (Chapter 1) through to the anti-science faith-based approach of Richard Hittleman (Chapter 12). In fact, these influences have travelled in two directions, with elements of European traditionalism penetrating yoga's heartland in North America.

In this book, I focus on the Anglo-American roots of modern postural practice, and in particular the fascistic and conspiratorial turns the ideologies associated with this type of yoga have taken over the past century. More specifically, the book traces the development of modern postural yoga in North America and Europe through the twentieth century, up to its explosion in popularity in the 1970s. As will become apparent, guru lineages have been repeatedly falsified in an attempt to make it appear as though modern yoga originated on the Indian subcontinent and is an ancient, rather than a recently invented, tradition. Much of the hype around yoga leans on cognitive priming: the deep cerebral desire we all have to see what we expect – or hope – to see. Just as fascism provides false solutions to real problems, those marketing modern postural practice have often relied on a cynical exploitation of human needs.

In short, the genesis and history of modern postural practice is deeply entangled with both occultism and the far right. To start building a credible history of yoga and its connections to fascism and occultism, it is therefore necessary to begin by unpacking its false history.

PART I

Happy Baby: A Grubby Guru Takes Us All to the Cleaners

Pierre Bernard (c.1875–1955) – portrayed by some as a key figure in spreading the Indian yogic tradition in the West – was a self-styled American yogi who liked to tell tall tales about his life. He was such an inveterate liar that it's hard to say for sure where he came from, although his biographer, Robert Love (who has a similar disregard for the facts and will be discussed further below) claims he was born in Leon, Iowa, on 31 October 1876. This supposed 'fact' is verified by Love with a claim that a relative of Bernard saw it inscribed in a family Bible. Bernard himself asserted he was born everywhere, from Chicago to Paris via Des Moines.

Bernard first came to widespread public attention in 1898 via press coverage reporting he performed a carnival trick involving slowing his breathing so that a doctor could insert surgical needles through his earlobes, cheek, upper lip and nostrils. This was hyped as a death trance in which the activity of the lungs and heart were lowered alongside body temperature, creating the illusion of death. Not bad as a sideshow act if the press stories are to be believed, but it failed to lift Bernard to the heights of fame enjoyed by escapologist Harry Houdini.

By the early twentieth century, Bernard's interests are reported to have shifted to teaching hypnotism and sexual practices. Around 1905, he founded the Tantrik Order of America somewhere on the West Coast – exactly where is disputed – although in reality this may have consisted of little more than Bernard telling people it existed. Bernard appears to have had an itinerant lifestyle at the time, and this shadowy organisation may have manifested itself as part of a travelling medicine show, popping up in towns all the way from Washington State down to California.

Bernard eventually shifted his base of operations to New York, where he focused on teaching a postural practice grounded in Western physical culture. In 1910, his name was splashed across the front pages of the press when he was charged with kidnapping two teenage girls, Zella Hopp and Gertrude Leo. He faced further charges including impersonating a medic, allegedly so that he could persuade Hopp to have sex with him as a cure for her weak heart. The New York press of the time, not knowing the standard spelling of the chanted word 'om', dubbed Bernard 'The Great Oom'.

After a compendium of tantric texts Bernard had slung together was dug up by a journalist, the papers carried salacious tales of sex rites, orgies and necromancy among the Tantrik Order of America. As the months went by and the kidnap case ground to a halt due to witnesses refusing to testify, the press lost interest. Whether or not the charges were dropped is disputed, but there doesn't seem to have been a final verdict on them.

Whatever its origins, by this time the Tantrik Order was an occult fraternity that might be seen as a smaller-scale sibling to the Theosophical Society or the Hermetic Order of the Golden Dawn. All drew ostentatiously, although often superficially, on Eastern spiritual beliefs, which they then proceeded to blend with Western esoteric thought and practices. What differentiated Bernard's order from the older operations was his greater stress on exercise. Nonetheless, those joining the group supposedly signed their names in blood on a Tantric Order contract, a carny stunt that would be repeated by later money-grabbing occult operations such as The Church of Satan.

Bernard carried on teaching what he called 'tantra' and 'yoga', but his practices seem to bear little relationship to what these words signify on the Indian subcontinent. His yoga, for instance, seems to have drawn more from Western physical culture than Eastern meditation. Even so, Bernard apparently charged top dollar for his services, with a good chunk of these fees successfully invested in real estate.

As the First World War drew to a close, heiress Margaret Stuyvesant Rutherfurd joined the yoga classes run by Bernard's wife, the dancer Blanche de Vries. Rutherfurd was carefully cultivated first by de Vries and later by Bernard. Rutherfurd's mother had married into the wealthy Vanderbilt family two years after being widowed, making Margaret a Vanderbilt stepchild. Eventually much of the family and their ultra-rich New York society friends were drawn into Bernard's circle, and from 1922 until 1929 Margaret was married to Bernard's British disciple Sir Paul Henry Dukes.

With the conclusion of the war, Bernard was in a position to set up what would become the Clarkstown Country Club in Nyack, New York, well away from the bustle of Manhattan. Once Bernard's Nyack operation was up and running, he was able to settle down into semi-respectability and pursue more lucrative business interests than yoga. These included becoming president of a bank and investing in an airport, dog-racing tracks and baseball stadiums. Bernard was also able to indulge himself by, among other things, having performing elephants stabled at his country club.

In short, once he'd amassed considerable wealth, Bernard became a stereotypical well-fed cigar-chomping capitalist. Perhaps it is Bernard's flash lifestyle and his connections to the ultra-high net-worth Vanderbilt set that has dazzled some of the journalists who have recently written mythological histories of 'jazz age' yoga in North America.

As we will see, the journalist most responsible for the faulty picture many now have of Bernard is the previously mentioned Robert Love, who toiled at American music paper *Rolling Stone* for 20 years, working his way up from researcher to managing editor before losing his job in 2002 amid falling sales and flatlining advertising revenue.[1] Given the many ways Love has amplified falsehoods about Bernard, he has become an integral part of this fake guru's story and the mythologising of modern yoga's origins.

1

Did Pierre Bernard Invent Yoga in California at the Start of the Twentieth Century?

The term 'yoga' refers to both a physical culture system that is slightly more than a century old and a set of religious practices whose origins pre-date those of postural yoga, though they were reinvented in the late nineteenth century. While the most well-known branch of modern postural yoga, which draws on Western physical culture and gained momentum in India in the 1920s, is reasonably well served research-wise,[1] the strand that runs from Pierre Bernard through the likes of Blanche de Vries, Clara Spring, Francis Yeats-Brown and Paul Dukes, is less well documented in terms of credible, verifiable information.

When it comes to modern yoga, sources cross and blend across continents. Although Pierre Bernard was American and taught in the US, two of his best-known disciples – Yeats-Brown and Dukes – were British, and their yogic activities had a huge impact in the UK, as well as other parts of the English-speaking world. Likewise, the culturally hybrid India-centred branch of yoga practice had a massive impact in North America, Australia, Latin America, and finally the whole Spanish-speaking world and elsewhere, through Indra Devi and others.[2]

What is fascinating about Bernard in particular is that he seems to have been teaching modern postural practice very early on in the game, possibly by 1905 and certainly within five years of this date. So did Bernard invent the postural yoga practice he taught, or did he learn it from someone else? The answer given by Robert Love in his biography *The Great Oom: The Improbable Birth of Yoga in America* is that Bernard learnt everything he knew from a guru called Sylvais Hamati. How does Love arrive at this position? According to the book's footnotes, his knowledge of the matter is entirely derived from his biographical subject, despite Bernard being shown in Love's account and elsewhere to be an unreliable source of information about both himself and his activities. Love begins Chapter 1 of his book as follows:

> Like most self-made men, Pierre Bernard was never at ease with the facts of his origins. Asked where he was born, he ... never, ever [volunteered] Leon, Iowa. Leon, the provincial capital of Decatur Country, was the true and actual birthplace of the Omnipotent Oom, who arrived in this world as Perry Arnold Baker in the year of America's centennial, 1876. This small town of 1,300 souls never measured up to Bernard's inflated sense of himself. 'May be alright to die in, but never thought much of it as a place in which to live,' he wrote to his cousin Martha Hoffman.[3]

As noted previously, Love's 'proof' of Bernard's place and date of birth is less than satisfactory, especially since this journalist knows the data is disputed.[4] Likewise, Love is not the first author to state that Bernard faked his own biography. Hugh B. Urban writes in his essay 'The Omnipotent Oom': 'Virtually nothing is known about the enigmatic Bernard's early life and background in fact, [*sic*] he seems to have gone to some lengths to conceal his real background behind a strange veil of fictitious identities and false biography, often using the fake persona of "Peter Coons" from Iowa.'[5]

Love, having established that Bernard is an unreliable 'witness', nevertheless proceeds – if his footnoting is to be believed – to rely pretty much exclusively on Bernard for his information about Sylvais Hamati:

> It is a maxim among spiritual seekers that when the student is ready, the teacher will appear. And so, as if plucked from a candlelit cave in the foothills of the Himalayas and materialized on the muddy streets of the frontier town of Lincoln, this dapper Asian émigré stood before the skinny, wide-eyed kid from Iowa. The odds against this meeting are not just long, they are nigh impossible; fewer than eight hundred Indians in total immigrated to the United States between 1820 and 1900 ...
>
> Hamati came to America from Calcutta, and may have arrived in the United States as a freelance tutor or an entertainer in a traveling show ... When they were introduced in a park in Lincoln, Perry was barely into his teens ... From that day on, Perry Baker [Pierre Bernard's birth name according to Love] would remain under Hamati's tutelage for eighteen years, working directly with him for up to three hours a day, diligently pursuing the exact course of study Hamati proposed ... .[6]

If this reads like fiction, that's because it appears to be so far removed from the facts that it fails to even hit the mark as 'new journalism'. Depending on which source one uses – and they may all be wrong – Hamati had a Persian or Syrian father and a French or Bengali mother. In other words, even if Hamati actually existed, he may not have been Indian/Asian.

Despite there being good reason to doubt almost anything Bernard said, Love later quotes – without any disclaimers – from the transcript of an interview Oom gave in which he asserts he was with Hamati 'continually' until he was 23 or 24.[7] Once we unravel Love's sources, it becomes apparent there has been no cross-checking of material about Hamati.[8] The book's footnotes for this section include sources that, while providing some relevant background material, don't explicitly mention Bernard's alleged guru. Moreover, the sources that do actually mention Hamati are limited to a deposition made by Bernard, notes made by Bernard, a quote from Bernard in a 1955 newspaper article, and a publication issued by an organisation run by Bernard.

To make matters worse, Love's 'independent' and 'cross-referenced' verification material is an interview in the 'IJTO'. Nowhere in his book does Love explain what these initials stand for, but it seems they are an abbreviation of *International Journal: Tantrick Order*.[9] Checking this publication – undated, circa 1906 – I found D. J. Elliott's interview with Swami Ram Tirath on pages 93 to 95. The main point of the feature appears to be to buttress and boost Bernard's status as head of the Tantrik Order of America. In the interview, Elliott asks 'What is your opinion of the American Primate Bernard, and how does he compare with the Tantrik High Priests of India?', to which Swami Ram Tirath replies: 'He is most earnest, sincere, and zealous for the cause; more energetic, and his knowledge just as extensive.'[10]

Swami Ram Tirath was a legitimate monk, but whether this interview is genuine is another matter entirely. It appears possible that D. J. Elliott was one of Bernard's pseudonyms, and even if it wasn't, it would seem that Oom – as the publisher and probably the editor of the journal – was in a position to manipulate the content of this 'interview'. In short, as a source of factual information about Pierre Bernard – and/or his alleged guru – the interview cannot reasonably be viewed as reliable.

Not only are Love's claims about Hamati taken from a single source (Bernard himself), which even he knows is unreliable, they don't add up. If Hamati actually existed and had studied tantra under a master in India for 19 years as claimed by Love via Bernard, why would he help put together such a typically Western occult publication of the *fin de siècle* as the *IJTO*? Even from Love's description of the contents – let alone looking at the actual journal – it seems highly unlikely that a student and his guru who between them had spent several decades diligently mastering traditional Indian/Bengali tantra would throw together a mishmash that seems to owe more to Christian missionary distortions of tantra than to its actual practice on the Indian subcontinent.

The fact that *The Great Oom* opts to depict Hamati as an 'Indian' (despite Love apparently knowing this may not be the case), tells us more about the prejudices of the author – and what he perceives to be the desires of his audience – than it does about the elusive and possibly non-existent guru. Since those attracted to 'embodied spirituality' are prone to fantasising that modern postural yoga originated in ancient India – rather than (as seems more likely) with nineteenth-century occidental circus acts and gymnastics – Love obligingly provides his readership with a wobbly portrayal of Hamati as an Indian-cum-Syrian: 'At their lodge at 1411A Golden Gate Avenue, snitches told the press, there was a dark skinned "turbanned Syrian"– Hamati, no doubt – who made frequent appearances.'[11]

Describing Bernard's first big media splash, when he put himself into a trance state and allowed needles to be passed through his skin, Love states: 'Hamati, who was not there that night physically, had taught him well. Bernard lengthened his respiration, slowed it, stretched it, thinned it to near nothing .... '[12] It is difficult to know if Hamati was ever physically 'there'. Perhaps he was just a figment of Bernard's imagination, or else an occidental sidekick who'd been told to wear a turban to impress those who shelled out money to participate in 'tantrik' activities.

Love's various dubious assertions about Hamati and Bernard have had profound consequences for how the history of modern yoga has been depicted since the turn of the millennium. Looking for information about Hamati often involves going around in circles and coming back to Love, and ultimately Bernard as his biographer's source of information on this phantom guru. Take, for example, the sources Stefanie Syman – who we will return to below – draws on in writing about Bernard and Hamati in her book, *The Subtle Body: The Story of Yoga In America*.[13] On inspection, Bernard emerges as the only individual mentioned in her notes who actually makes direct claims to have met Hamati. Meanwhile, Paul G. Hackett, whose dissertation Syman cites, later wrote the book *Theos Bernard, The White Lama: Tibet, Yoga, and American Religious Life*, in which he makes clear that his information about Hamati comes from Robert Love.[14] Religious studies academic Jeffrey J. Kripal also credits his information about Hamati to Robert Love in the footnotes to his essay *Remembering Ourselves*.[15]

Much remains uncertain about Bernard, including his original name and date of birth. Academic Hugh B. Urban is as flummoxed about the details of Bernard's life as Love or Syman, but unlike them he signals his uncertainty.[16] Urban also suggests Bernard's tantric practice was an occidental reinvention of Indian subcontinent traditions fused with Western sex magic, rather than a continuation of ancient practices. Indeed, it was Bernard's sexual teachings and the media scandals connected to them that attracted the extensive press coverage he received in the early part of the twentieth century.

As might be deduced from Hugh Urban's description of his tantra, Bernard's postural yoga can be seen as a modern

Western invention spiced up with a smattering of Sanskrit terms. Even Syman appears to reluctantly recognise this – at least to some extent – when she writes:

> Yoga could still use some help. 'The Yogi's [Bernard's] teaching was a pleasing mixture of Couéism, Childs dietetics, first aid to the injured, mysticism, and Bernarr Macfadden, combining the best features of each,' wrote E. B. White in *The New Yorker* in March 1928.
>
> White had captured the essence of American yoga of the era. Hatha Yoga postures did resemble elements of Macfadden's physical culture. And the vocabulary of New Thought that permeated contemporary presentations of yoga, including Bernard's, undeniably echoed Émile Coué's autosuggestion.[17]
>
> It wasn't so much the content of yoga that White got wrong as the efficacy and coherence of the discipline. No one seemed to believe that these techniques taken together amounted to much or could be part of a meaningful philosophy – with its own metaphysics and theology.[18]

As the last paragraph of the above implies, Syman appears unable to accept that modern yoga is merely a bricolage of mostly occidental elements, and instead attempts to construct an ancient Indian lineage for the practice. In his book *Yoga Body*, Mark Singleton details the origin of much postural yoga in Western exercise systems, but to these it appears we must add circus acrobatics and stage magic. Love even mentions in passing that, like Harry Houdini, Bernard 'found a lucrative niche making his knowledge of magic and illusion for sale to debunkers and scientific sceptics'.[19] Bernard's immersion in circus and magic tricks offers a pointer to where much of his yoga comes from, perhaps buttressed by the dance exercises of his wife and other female disciples.

Those like Love and Syman who endorse Bernard's claims about his guru lineage actively avoid acknowledging the possibility that modern postural practice essentially sprang into being on the West Coast of America at the start of the twentieth century, when Oom and those around him bolted colonialist interpretations of traditions hailing from the Indian subcontinent onto the Western physical culture of the period. Understandings of tantra and yoga had, by the time they reached Bernard's circle, become interwoven with Christianity, European occultism and New Thought. While little of what Bernard and his circle said and did was original to them, they were – as far as we know – the first group of people to bring these elements together under the rubric of 'yoga'. As such, modern yoga can be considered, at least partly, a twentieth-century occidental confabulation with some orientalist fairy dust sprinkled on top, in a desperate attempt to justify the frequently made claim it can be traced back thousands of years to the Indus Valley.

2
The Great Oom and White Power

Unlike his follower, the notorious British fascist Francis Yeats-Brown, Bernard does not appear to have been an enthusiastic fan of Hitler and the Nazis or Mussolini's corporatist ideology. Bernard comes across as having been far more interested in making money than changing the political set-up of North American and European countries. Nevertheless, Yeats-Brown was not the only white supremacist among Oom's followers – and it seems that Bernard himself shared their racist worldview. Certainly, he wasn't averse to endorsing works by his top disciples in which they espoused such views. In short, yoga and tantra were claimed as Aryan – that is, white – pursuits by Bernard's circle on the basis that the Hindu caste system was created to preserve racial purity in India and those of high caste were (at the inception of the system) Aryan. They shared this position with Nazi racial theorists.

In her PhD dissertation 'Yoga in America: History, Community Formation, and Consumerism' (subsequently issued as a book), Rebecca Anne D'Orsogna does a reasonable job of applying famous French theorist Michel Foucault's theories to the sexual aspects of Bernard's teachings and practice. She is less successful, however, when it comes to addressing issues around race.[1] In this respect, D'Orsogna follows Love in viewing journalist and Oom acolyte Hamish McLaurin's 1933 book *Eastern Philosophy For Western Minds* as 'an introduction to Bernard's version of Indian wisdom'.[2] After an introduction by Francis Yeats-Brown, McLaurin's text begins by arguing yoga is Aryan:

> Perhaps not one person out of ten thousand in the western world ever has heard of yoga, or, having heard of it, has the faintest conception of what it is. A few know of it as being an ancient system of self-culture which tends to lengthen life, promote health, build strength, and insure peace of mind and happiness. Even of that few, not all are aware that this time tested scheme for human betterment was devised by their own ancestors, the early Aryans, at least five thousand years ago ...
>
> One reason why the truths contained in the old Sanskrit writings are not more widely known and highly regarded in the West is that they have so long been identified with a people who differ from us in colour. Because the Indo-Aryan texts were treasured and preserved in India, it has been taken for granted that they were the product of a dark-skinned race. This, of course, is not true. They are, and always have been from a racial standpoint—the legitimate heritage of the peoples now in the ascendancy throughout Europe and the New World.[3]

Skipping forward to Chapter III, we find the racism of the Bernard circle even more blatantly articulated:

> The Aryans, when they arrived in India, were a highly developed race. They represented the purest possible white stock. Biologically they were the equals of any white race existing today, and there is every reason for the assumption that, in some of their faculties and capacities, they were our superiors. Therefore the moment they crossed the Indian frontier and encountered a dark-skinned people infinitely

beneath them on the evolutionary scale, they were confronted with a grave problem ... Having gained control over their dusky brethren through a superior knowledge of physical and mental phenomena, it was no part of the Aryan scheme to let the people of the lower castes have access to that knowledge until such time as they had evolved to a point at which they became capable of handling it. A scalpel may safely be entrusted to the hands of an expert surgeon. In the hands of a child it becomes a menace.[4]

Despite the racist ideology clearly on display in this tract, those writing about McLaurin's book in recent decades have generally chosen to skirt around it. Instead, they appear to be more interested in using the text to reinforce modern myths about Bernard, his disciples and yoga more broadly. Love, for instance, completely ignores the relationship some of Bernard's most prominent disciples have to racism and fascism, while D'Orsogna restricts herself to coyly hinting at such views by placing the words 'Indo-Aryan' in quote marks:

With Bernard's blessing, Hamish McLaurin, a student and 'stalwart member' of the CCC, attempted to convey Bernard's 'Indo-Aryan' teaching to Americans in *Eastern Philosophy for Western Minds* (1933), one of the first prescriptive American interpretations of Hatha yoga ... As a student of Bernard's, 'a promoter, an entrepreneur ... a public relations guy,' McLaurin adapted his teacher's understanding of how to explain yoga in a manner that would resonate with Americans. In this carefully crafted promotional work, McLaurin avoided precise detail regarding the physical aspects of yoga.[5]

What D'Orsogna describes as a 'carefully crafted promotional work' might equally be characterised as a racist rant designed to 'resonate' only with those Americans who self-identify as white.

The white supremacist ideology that permeates McLaurin's work can be traced all the way back to the 1906 edition of the Tantrik Order journal published and probably edited by Bernard, indicating that Oom's 'racialised elitism', as D'Orsogna terms it, had already bubbled to the surface during his earliest days in New York. To give just a couple of examples: 'The Tantras deal almost exclusively with the practical side of the Aryan Religion ... It is upon these arts and sciences that the Ancient Aryans depended for the accomplishment of all worldly desires' (p.9); and 'The bridge of thoughts and sighs that spans the whole history of the Aryan-World, has its first arch in the Veda' (p.10).[6]

Admittedly, the relevant passages are mostly not Bernard's own words, instead emerging from a collage of citations he published. Nevertheless, the manner in which they are deployed and the fact they appear in his journal indicates that they – by and large – reflect Bernard's own perspectives. Moreover, they mirror the views later espoused by McLaurin.

While the press may have framed Bernard as 'closer to Indian than white',[7] this is not how Bernard was perceived by at least some of his disciples, who, as unabashed white supremacists, saw him as Aryan. In McLaurin's case, it is clear that at least part of Bernard's appeal as a guru is that he promoted an Aryan ethical code supposedly based on tantra, which both men appear to have perceived as the true heritage of the 'white race'.

Perhaps if Bernard hadn't been able to attract disciples via newspaper coverage that depicted him as a quack and a charlatan – D'Orsogna highlights the Wertheim sisters as an example of heiresses seeking out the unsavoury Oom as a form of youthful rebellion – his brand of cod-spiritual yoga wouldn't have taken hold among those of a fascist and white supremacist bent. And perhaps if these unsavoury aspects of the Great Oom's philosophy hadn't been brushed over by more recent writers on the history of modern postural yoga, current exponents of the practice would have a more clear-sighted and less cult-like perspective on its century-old – rather than pan-millennia – origins. Sadly, neither has been the case, and the close intertwining of twentieth-century postural yoga with white supremacism remains little known among the public at large.

Nevertheless, better late than never, and with the aim of filling in the blanks, the next part of this book turns the spotlight on the various far-right yoga aficionados who followed in Bernard's wake.

PART II

Warrior One, Two and Three:
Fascism + Yoga = Fascist Yoga
(The 1920s to the 1940s)

Before fully immersing ourselves in the post-World War I world of fascist yoga, it is worthwhile pausing to discuss the role played by 'Yogi' Ramacharaka and notorious British occultist Aleister Crowley. Alongside Pierre Bernard, they are both key early figures in the development of modern occult yoga, and both owe a huge debt to Helena Blavatsky and her theosophy movement.

Yogi Ramacharaka was in reality William Walker Atkinson, an American New Thought proponent who used his Indian-sounding pseudonym to write extensively about Hinduism and yoga in the early twentieth century. *Hatha Yoga*, written under the Ramacharaka pen name and published in 1904, is considered by some to be the first modern book on hatha yoga. The fitness exercises it features are derived from Western physical culture but differ from the Scandinavian primitive gymnastics that around the same time – probably shortly afterwards – were being repackaged as yoga *asanas* (body postures).[1] Despite not matching classic modern postural practice in terms of its exercises, this 1904 work did help establish a template for later hatha yoga books, with sections on diet, breathing, relaxation, sleep, cleansing and workout.

Walker has left an imprint on the discourse that surrounds modern postural practice and in terms of fascist yoga, his influence is perhaps most evident on Ezra Pound (1885–1972). Pound was renowned for his poetry but notorious for his radio broadcasts supporting the Axis powers between 1941 and 1945. As a US citizen, Pound was charged with treason after the war, but found mentally unfit to stand trial. From the end of 1945 until May 1958, Pound was held in an American psychiatric hospital; when he was released, he returned to Italy, where he had lived from 1924 until his arrest.

While there has been copious scholarly debate about Pound's involvement with fascism, few academics have had much to say about his yoga practice and its impact on his worldview and poetry. One of those who does, Demetres P. Tryphonopoulos, identifies the primary source for Pound's yoga practice as Yogi Ramacharaka:

> ... a number of whose books appeared in the first decade of this century [i.e., the twentieth century], including *Fourteen Lessons in Yogi Philosophy* and *Oriental Occultism* (1903). In fact, Pound refers to this writer in a footnote to his 1908 sonnet 'Plotinus' (CEP 296) and to one of his books, *Hatha Yoga* ... in his poem 'Moeurs Contemporaines'.[2]

Tryphonopoulos also suggests that:

> It is possible that Pound is indebted to Ramacharaka's books for some of his occult ideas. For example, in *Fourteen Lessons* he could have encountered the concept of the 'subtle body', that is, belief in an order of existence which is not incorporeal but of an order of corporeality which cannot be perceived ordinarily.

It should be stressed that for reactionaries like Pound, yoga is not separate from but very much entwined with fascist activism. Thus, this fascist poet's white supremacist disciple John Kasper – a suspect in a school bombing in Nashville, as well as a number of synagogue bombings – was encouraged by his incarcerated mentor to set up the Make It New bookshop in Greenwich Village (which opened in 1953), and use it to propagate not just writing by Pound and those he admired, but also yoga.[3] In his book *John Kasper and Ezra Pound*, Alec Marsh writes:

> Yoga classes were among the shop's after hours offerings. Evidently, it was Pound who drafted the anti-dope message that was put on a sign outside the bookshop: 'Pot

smokers who want to quit. Correct use of breathing exercises described in these books will give you all the remarkable sensations you can get from marijuana anywhere ... The reds have been using drugs as a political weapon since 1932. Don't be a Rooseveltian dupe ... .'[4]

For Pound, yoga and its breathing techniques as taught by 'Ramacharaka' might not only save the world from drug addiction, but from what he perceived to be Communism. The other side of William Walker Atkinson's written output as a New Thought booster may have been of assistance to Pound in maintaining such delusional beliefs. Understanding human beings as possessing divinely powerful minds, New Thought, with its message that correct mental attitudes can overcome all difficulties in life – including debilitating illness – was a direct precursor to today's positive thinking.[5] More specifically, New Thought's insistence that by mentally accessing the infinite power of spirit it is possible to control the physical world can also be found in much yogic and occult discourse, including that woven around Aleister Crowley.

Crowley, although not politically a fascist, has been accused of fascist leanings. He appears to have been one of the first people to teach yoga in England, but adapted it for the Western world by combining it with the ceremonial magic he learned as a member of the Hermetic Order of the Golden Dawn. In *India And The Occult*, Gordan Djurdjevic describes how, from around 1907 onwards, Crowley used the occult orders he was involved with to propagate a mix of Western and Eastern esoteric practices, concluding that 'In its essence, the method of the A∴A∴ rests on the fusion of Western ceremonial magick and Yoga.'[6]

Aside from J. F. C. Fuller, discussed below, Crowley clearly influenced the ideas put forward in the pre-Second World War yoga books issued by UK publishing company Rider, and those written by bestselling yoga author Desmond Dunne later on. Given these writers were mostly seeking universal occult truths, they discarded much of the specifically Hindu/Indian subcontinent elements of Eastern esoteric practice. Likewise, Crowley's assessment of the extent to which the *Aphorisms of Patajañali* are useful clearly diminished between his *Book 4* (1912) and *Eight Lectures On Yoga*, published 27 years later:[7]

> The great classic of Sanskrit literature is the *Aphorisms of Patajañali*. He is at least mercifully brief, and not more than ninety or ninety-five percent of what he writes can be dismissed as the ravings of a disordered mind. What remains is twenty-four carat gold. I now proceed to bestow it.[8]

Crowley and the occult yoga practitioners who followed in his wake were interested in what they viewed as useful from the Eastern traditions they plundered. Keith Cantú puts it this way in his PhD, 'Sri Sabhapati Swami and the "Translocalization" of *Śivarājayoga*':

> ... a primary intent of some occult authors—at least as explicitly stated—was to learn and disseminate techniques that were deemed objectively efficacious, and not to intentionally exoticize or inscribe difference. This is perhaps most exemplified by the negative attitude towards 'Oriental' fascination with yoga in Crowley's *Eight Lectures on Yoga*.[9]

The prose of occultists in this tradition who weren't political fascists reads very differently to much of the writing by those involved with modern postural practice; the latter generally treat the decorative Hindu facade adorning their occidental gymnastic activities with great earnestness. Mirroring its Aryanism, there is in explicitly fascist yoga an orientalist lionising of supposed ancient Indo-European practices and spirituality that matches similar but less obviously racist tendencies on this score found in the less overtly occultist forms of modern postural practice.

My road to learning about fascist yoga was a long and winding one. When a handful of those I'd known on the London punk music scene of the late 1970s joined the far-right National Front and became countercultural fascists, I stopped speaking to them but began educating myself about their beliefs. Previously, some of those former friends had attended anti-racist events and gigs by multi-racial bands with me. As already mentioned, in 2016 I saw a newspaper profile of a yoga-practicing fascist. Once I started looking, it wasn't hard to identify other fascist yogis, both historical and contemporary. I was primed to seek out this information because the passive-aggressive behaviour of several yoga instructors I'd encountered and the unctuous bullshit they spouted had left me feeling completely hacked off.

Pierre Bernard's circle may have been stuffed to the gills with white supremacists from the get go, but it wasn't until the mid-1920s that a full-blown mystical fascist in the form of Francis Yeats-Brown — aka the 'Bengal Lancer' — joined the Nyack gang. Before that, a group of far-right Italians got their fascist yoga groove going when in 1920 nudist and group sex enthusiast Guido Keller produced a swastika-emblazoned publication called *YOGA* to indulge his absurdist avant-garde inclinations.[10] More buttoned-up than Keller was the previously mentioned British fascist Major J. F. C. Fuller, who bizarrely applied some of the occult dreck he'd learned from Crowley to his extensive writings on warfare. Other notable names from this era — all of whom will be scrutinised in greater detail below — include the Nazi Indologist and religious studies writer Jakob Wilhelm Hauer, self-styled Italian 'super-fascist' Julius Evola, far-right activist Savitri Devi (born Maximiani Portas to an English mother of Italian descent and a French father of Greek descent), and Romanian 'intellectual' and fiction writer Mircea Eliade.

Before delving deeper into the murky lives and beliefs of these various far-right yoga enthusiasts, it is important to make the point that fascist ideology is today often over-identified with Hitler's National Socialist German Workers Party (*Nationalsozialistische Deutsche Arbeiterpartei* – NSDAP) regime in Germany during the 1930s and 1940s. While all Nazis are fascists, not all fascists are necessarily Nazis – even within Germany's post-First World War milieu, the NSDAP was merely the most successful force among a number of competing fascist and far-right groups. Likewise, within the NSDAP, there was a diversity of opinion not only as to whether Indo-German (aka neo-Hindu) or other beliefs (including both Norse and Christian faiths) constituted a better religious basis for fascism, but whether the primary focus should be placed on the 'nationalist' or the 'socialist' element within so-called 'National Socialism'. These sometimes conflicting opinions are reflected in the views of the fascist yoga practitioners presented in the following chapters, each of which have, in their own way, influenced the evolution of (at least certain strands of) modern postural yoga.

3
Guido Keller and the Rijeka Yoga Group

In *The Birth of Fascist Ideology*,[1] Zeev Sternhell suggests this political creed first emerged in France in 1913. While there is ongoing debate around the accuracy of his conclusions, we can take this date as marking – at least roughly – the start of the period in which fascist yoga was soon to appear. If fascism as an ideology emerged in France, it first developed as a mass movement in Italy. Given the attraction certain strands of fascism hold for yoga – both in neo-Hindu and other guises – and the occult, it comes as little surprise that a group called YOGA was active around what was perhaps the first attempt to create a fascist state: namely, the Italian Regency of Carnaro.

After the First World War, there were disputes over the status of the city of Rijeka (called Fiume in Italian), and on 12 September 1919, the Italian poet and far-right military 'hero' Gabriele D'Annunzio (1863–1938) led a rag-tag army of fascist legionnaires into the seaport and announced he had annexed it for Italy. Rather than accepting this, the not-yet-fascist Italian state attempted to blockade the city in line with the wishes of the then dominant international order – or more specifically the victorious allies of the First World War. Nevertheless, D'Annunzio held onto the city and on 8 September 1920 declared it an independent state with a corporatist – that is, fascist – Constitution. Selflessly, he appointed himself at its head.

WARRIOR ONE, TWO AND THREE: FASCISM + YOGA = FASCIST YOGA

D'Annunzio has the reputation of being both the 'John The Baptist of fascism' and a 'cocaine-snorting, bed-hopping egomaniac'.[2] His brief dictatorship in Rijeka created the forms of choreographed far-right spectacle that Benito Mussolini and later Hitler appropriated:

> Virtually the entire ritual of Fascism came from the 'Free State of Fiume': the balcony address, the Roman salute, the cries of 'aia, aia, alala,' the dramatic dialogues with the crowd, the use of religious symbols in a new secular setting, the eulogies to the 'martyrs' of the cause and the employment of their 'relics' in political ceremonies. Moreover, quite aside from the poet's contribution to the form and style of Fascist politics, Mussolini's movement first started to attract great strength when the future dictator supported D'Annunzio's occupation of Fiume.[3]

D'Annunzio also claimed to be the greatest Italian writer since Dante. Like Bernard, he had little time for the truth and created a fake biography for himself. One story told about D'Annunzio is that he had his lower ribs removed so that he could bend far enough forward to perform fellatio on himself. While this rib removal tale may or may not be true, it seems all-too-apt given his increasingly monstrous narcissism. This fascistic, self-regarding inward turn – also observable in more recent right-wing figures like Donald Trump – can perhaps be seen as reflecting the yogic obsession with personal transformation at the expense of genuine social change.

D'Annunzio's confidant and political enforcer in Rijeka was Guido Keller (1892–1929), who like his boss was a decorated fighter pilot and dandy. Keller was also notorious as a manic depressive, with his mental instability not particularly helped by his copious use of cocaine. Described as D'Annunzio's 'freelance quartermaster and morale booster' by scholar John Woodhouse,[4] Keller is said to have organised the hijacking of the trucks to convey his superior's legionnaires to Rijeka. Moreover, it has also been claimed that he personally flew around the Adriatic seeking to plunder whatever supplies couldn't be stolen from the population directly under fascist control.[5]

Keller formed the YOGA group with Giovanni Comisso (1895–1969), who went on to become a literary figure admired by parts of Italy's bourgeois cultural establishment. The Futurist Mino Somenzi also belonged to YOGA. In fact, YOGA was both an outgrowth of and reaction to the cultural-cum-political Futurist movement led by F. T. Marinetti, who as early as 1909 celebrated war as 'the world's only hygiene', and later became a high-profile fascist. Revisionist historian Günter Berghaus – whose research appears to be sound in places, although the conclusions he draws from it are ludicrous – relates that:

> After Marinetti's and Vecchi's departure, Mario Carli and Mino Somenzi took over the leadership of the Futurist flock in Fiume. Keller, whom Marinetti had praised in his diary as a true *futurista*, became a close friend and collaborator. This Fascio Futurista Fiumanese founded a newspaper, *La testa di ferro*, edited by Mario Carli, whose first number appeared on 1 February 1920. Keller called into existence a group called YOGA, which ran a regular column in *La testa di ferro* and for a short period also published their own journal: *Yoga: Unione di spiriti liberi tendenti alla perfezione* (November to December 1920).[6]

While D'Annunzio wasn't – as far as can be gleaned – an official member of the new group, the 'theoretical' aspects of YOGA appear to have drawn heavily on his writing and ideas. It has also been claimed the purpose of YOGA was to protect

D'Annunzio from the influence of the arch-conservatives who supported him, with Keller, Comisso and Somenzi viewing these reactionaries as too moderate for their fascist tastes.[7]

Those involved in YOGA were all fascinated by orientalised versions of mysticism — hence their name, and possibly one of the reasons for their use of the swastika. A favoured activity of the group was to gather under a fig tree in the square next to the house they occupied. Here, they indulged themselves with improvised fascist theatre, singing, dancing and drawing on the walls of buildings, while trying to lure passersby into debates on subjects such as free love. Along this vein, the *Strange History* blog describes the group as follows:

> Many of the YOGA club specialized in the red lotus: they became ecstatics, confirming themselves in extreme experiences of the senses, sex chief among them. Others were brown lotuses, tree-hugging and at times, you have the sense, ready to rip the tree from the ground to bring it down on the head of the enemy. All talked constantly of freedom, but only the exceptional would ever enjoy that freedom.[8]

On the one hand, YOGA purportedly rejected race in favour of a spiritual hierarchy drawn along 'traditional' Indo-European (aka neo-Hindu lines) — as the *Strange History* blog describes it: 'It wanted to borrow a caste system from the Hindus but it wanted to separate humans out not according to their genetic descent but rather according to their spiritual potential: the eugenics of karma, let's call it.' On the other hand, it still managed to extol racial nationalism — like many of today's fascists, fanning the flames of selected nationalist disputes. In YOGA's case, these included taking sides against the British Empire, which meant supporting both Indian and Irish nationalism, alongside support for more local struggles that would benefit Italy. YOGA's short-lived weekly publication, which was decorated with a 'life-giving' swastika and a five-petalled rose, argued that 'the genius of the Italian race' had been 'perverted by the democratic and bourgeois ideas of the "negative races", English, French and above all Jews'.[9]

YOGA wanted to restore Italy to greatness by returning the bulk of its citizens to traditional occupations. The Constitution of the short-lived regime they supported had nine corporations representing the different sectors of the conventional economy and employment. The members of YOGA, however, presumably saw themselves as belonging to the tenth corporation, which was reserved for 'superior individuals' ('poets', 'heroes' and 'supermen' – that is, D'Annunzio and anyone he favoured). Membership of a corporation was compulsory, with the Carta del Carnaro – which also designated music as the fundamental principle of the state – laying this down as law (although the Carta was never put into practice).

Taking a closer look at the politics of the YOGA group members, in analysing one of Giovanni Comisso's books, Derek Duncan observes that:

> The programme set out was hardly unique: the scathing attack on the bourgeois Italian state blames all of the nation's ills on contamination by 'other races' ... The call for national renewal is staged through a rejection of modernity ... The whole is tinged with imperial ambition ... Fiume offers Comisso a space for the production of homosexual desire that finds its justification in imperial domination and national renewal.[10]

Like Ernst Jünger (author of Hitler's favourite book *Storms of Steel*) and Francis Yeats-Brown (see Chapter 5), Comisso's early writing was informed by his experiences in the military. His first book of prose – *Il porto dell'amore* (*The Seaport of Love*, 1924) – was a collection of stories based on his experiences as a participant in D'Annunzio's occupation of Rijeka. Another similarity between the three writers is that Comisso's admirers continue to claim he wasn't a fascist on the basis that he didn't join Mussolini's Fascisti, just as Jünger never joined the NSDAP and Yeats-Brown wasn't a member of the British Union of Fascists. While little of Comisso's work is available in English, this passage about Rijeka from *Le mie stagioni* (*My Seasons*) can be found online:

> Guido Keller told me that he had just formed a company to guard the Commander, a company that he called *La Disperata* ['The Desperate'] ... These new soldiers spent most of the day swimming or rowing, or singing and marching through the city, bare-chested and dressed in shorts. They were not obliged to stay in the barracks ... and in the evening they frequented a deserted area called La torretta, where they split into two groups and did battle with real hand grenades, often leading to injury ... The presence of a number of morally dubious elements did not sully the company's reputation, but rather gave it the crepuscular flavour of a group despised by the wise and the mediocre, and this was its greatest source of pride.[11]

The Desperate used the slogan '*me ne frego*' ('I don't give a damn'), which was later taken up by Mussolini's fascists, and were sometimes called 'the soldiers of death', having cultivated a reputation for cruelty. The following description of Keller and Rijeka by Reinaldo Laddaga is far from unique in being overly romantic:

> ... curious war hero Guido Keller ... was one of the new commander's main lieutenants. The universe around the leader quickly fragmented into factions. Forced to take sides, D'Annunzio came to rely mostly on the young artists,

anarchists, and arditi who constituted the radical wing of the grand alliance of Fiume, and who formed the 'Union of Free Spirits Tending Toward Perfection' (or, as they nicknamed it, 'Yoga'). The group shared an enthusiasm for Hinduism, spiritual aristocracy, nudism, and for building an agrarian utopia where preindustrial forms of life would be restored.[12]

For YOGA, philosophy wasn't 'love of wisdom' but rather 'wisdom of love'. The group developed ideas around a 'science of love' as a means of transfiguration. Comisso is described by some sources as having a yogic background, and went on to write about India among other things, but it remains unclear whether any members of the group he co-founded actually practiced postural yoga. Nevertheless, regardless of whether Keller and company engaged in headstands, their liberal use of a cod-spirituality that drew on Hinduism, together with a fascistic attitude to physical and mental perfection, demonstrates the group were very much in the mould of the later postural yoga cults that were to emerge around the world.

The YOGA group are an early example of countercultural fascism. That said, many will find more significance in the way attempts to rehabilitate Keller, Comisso, YOGA and D'Annunzio, are tied to twenty-first-century culture wars. The YOGA group are mentioned in Aidan O'Malley's essay 'The Fascist Precursor', but what he's mainly interested in doing is weighing rival exhibitions in Rijeka and Trieste on the hundredth anniversary of D'Annunzio's occupation against Dominique Kirchner Reill's book *The Fiume Crisis: Life in the Wake of the Habsburg Empire*.

Of the Trieste show O'Malley says: 'Instead of offering critical insight into d'Annunzio or Fiume, this exhibition vigorously burnished the myth, and was little more than a city-sponsored display of a fetish ... .' By way of contrast, the same author says of the Rijeka exhibition that it:

> ... did not present *l'impresa di Fiume* as an idealised poetic endeavour, but as a brutal political act that directly impinged on the lives of people in the city ... d'Annunzio could perhaps be seen as a prototype for politicians like Berlusconi and Trump whose frankly improbable assertions of virility ... do little more than highlight their unearned sense of entitlement.[13]

As O'Malley notes in his essay, there were also diplomatic exchanges between Croatia and Italy over the erection of a statue of D'Annunzio in Trieste on the hundredth anniversary of the occupation of Rijeka. While statues and museum displays often play a leading role in contemporary culture wars, the republication of the four issues of the *YOGA* paper in a 2019 book should not be overlooked. This is *Yoga. Sovversivi e rivoluzionari con d'Annunzio a Fiume* by Simonetta Bartolini, which the publisher promoted with the following words:

> A revolution in the name of poetry, beauty, popular self-determination, and the supremacy of spirit over matter should have started in Fiume ... In this book Simonetta Bartolini reconstructs the history of 'Yoga' and the movement of the same name born in the 'city of life' in the summer of 1920, of the difficult relationship between Comisso and Keller with the beloved/hated d'Annunzio, tracing a meticulous interpretative path that – outside the pro-futurist or even pre-1968 cliché – finally places this piece of the intellectuals' humanism back in the correct historical perspective ... .[14]

Bartolini might be understood to be using the correct historical perspective according to Italian culture war ideology, but this is not a viewpoint everyone shares. It certainly isn't one Jonathan Bousfield has much time for, when he writes:

> What's important is that D'Annunzio was a leading proponent of an unashamedly Latin imperialism that saw Slavs as a lesser culture, that he regarded military takeovers as superior to diplomacy, and that he saw the alchemic pseudo-democracy of popular acclaim as superior to any electoral parliamentary system.
>
> The revisionism of today's Dannunzians doesn't just serve to legitimize the takeover of Rijeka in 1919, it also legitimizes Hitler's takeover of Austria in 1938, the Serbian rebel takeover of the Kraijina in 1990–91, or indeed Vladimir Putin's foisting of war upon the Donbas in 2014.[15]

The attempt to rehabilitate the likes of D'Annunzio and the Rijeka YOGA group is just one small part of a hybrid war being waged by the right in an attempt to replace the democratic norms of the latter part of the twentieth century with the 'might is right ideology' of fascism. While those participating in such revisionism object to their heroes being called fascists, self-proclaimed neo-Nazis also celebrate D'Annunzio and those associated with the Rijeka YOGA group.[16]

Ultimately, both YOGA and the Italian Regency of Carnaro disappeared as a consequence of the approval of the Treaty of Rapallo on 12 November 1920, which turned the territory into an independent state under international law: the *Slobodna Država Rijeka/Stato libero di Fiume* (Free State of Rijeka/Fiume). At first, D'Annunzio refused to leave the city, but his legionnaires – including the YOGA group – were forced out after being bombarded by Italian forces during the 1920 Christmas holiday.

4

Military Theorist Major J. F. C. Fuller, Whose Concept of Blitzkrieg Became Standard Practice in Nazi Warfare

During the inter-war years, two prominent British fascists published books on yoga: Major J. F. C. Fuller (1878–1966) and Major Francis Yeats-Brown (the latter of whom is addressed in the following chapter). Both men learned the bulk of their yoga at the feet of elitist occidental occultists who they accepted as 'masters'. However, rather than 'fessing up to the real sources of their practice, each attempted to deceive the public into believing they'd learned their smarts in India.

Fuller – known as 'Boney' due to his admiration for Napoleon Bonaparte – had a reasonably high-flying army career until the early 1930s, but he was also a well-known military historian whose interest in armoured warfare led him to develop the idea of the 'blitzkrieg', a tactic that would later be deployed to full effect by the Nazi regime. Fuller was a top member of the British Union of Fascists and also implicated in plots to overthrow the UK government and replace it with a puppet Nazi regime. In 1935, Boney was accorded the dubious privilege of being invited to witness Germany's first armed manoeuvres since Hitler's NSDAP had ascended to power. This paled in comparison, however, to being made guest of honour at the enormous three-hour motorised military parade that formed the centrepiece of the Führer's fiftieth birthday celebrations on 20 April 1939.

Turning to the genealogy of Fuller's yoga system, which seems to be have been inspired by another unsavoury individual decades previously, historian Kate Imy has done much of the archival spadework:[1]

> His published works maintained that as a soldier in India he studied 'the Vedas and the Upanishads' and 'took a deep interest in the Yoga philosophy' after meeting 'holy men, yogis, advanced radicals ... and various members of the Arya Samaj' ... however, Fuller's unpublished letters and diaries suggest that his immersion in yoga came less from conversing with unnamed Indian leaders than through his connections to the British occult. While sick with enteric fever in Lucknow in 1905, he read the poetic works of occultist and magician Aleister Crowley.[2]

Fuller soon became one of Crowley's disciples. Perhaps the greatest expression of Boney's love for his notorious yoga/occult guru can be found in his book *The Star in the West: A Critical Essay Upon the Works of Aleister Crowley*,[3] which reveals that the latter had already impressed his views on this particular student nearly twenty years before the *chela* (disciple) wrote his first and only full book on yoga:

> How is this inward mystery revealed? And the answer is: In the East by Yoga, and in the West by Magic ... In the East, by an entirely artificial and scientific method, in the West by a stimulation and sudden outflowing of the poetic faculty. The East, we may take it, is almost entirely static; whilst the West is wholly dynamic. Yet their methods, whatever they may be, ultimately harmonize (as everything ultimately must do), leading the aspirant through various stages of

illuminism, till he stands out from the illusions of his birth, and becomes one with that higher glow of glory in exalted states of Ecstasy or Samadhi.[4]

Fuller and Crowley eventually fell out circa 1910, seemingly over Crowley's indulgence in sex magic with other men, and indifference to defending his reputation when his masculinity was questioned as a result. Before this break, however, Boney spent half a decade operating as both his master's cheerleader and his hatchet-man against rivals (including Indian yogis). An example of the latter role can be seen in the satirical sketch, 'Half-Hours With Famous Mahatmas No. 1', that Fuller wrote for Crowley's journal *The Equinox:*[5]

'Do you know Swami Vivekananda?' I asked.

'Ha,' he replied, 'he no good, he my disciple, I am the master!'

'And Swami Dayanand Sarasvati?' I continued. The same answer was vouched to me, although this latter teacher had died at the age of seventy, forty years ago. Thinking it about time to change the conversation, I said: 'O Thou Shower from the Highest! Tell thy grovelling disciple what then "is" a "lie"?'

'Ha!' he replied, 'it is illusion, this truth that has been diverged from its real point; an illusive spring in the primogenial fermentation of "fee-no-me-non," in this typocosmy apparent to the sense which you call "deVurld"!!!'

With this, and promises of oceans of blissful reality from the highest eternality of ultimate ecstasy, he bade me sit in a chair and blow alternately through my nostrils; and, if I had faith, so he assured me, I should in six months time arrive at the supreme stage of the Highest in the infinite Ultimatum, and should burst as a chance illusively fermented bubble in the purest atmosphere of the highest reality.

This Vedanta parody nods to Crowley's meeting with Mahatma Agamya Paramahamsa at around the time Fuller became his disciple, echoing press coverage of a 1908 court case in which the then 67-year-old Indian guru's attempts to run a patriarchal 'love cult' in West Hampstead (north London) resulted in a sentence of four months' hard labour for assault. It also prompted a lecture from the magistrate, who suggested that this reprobate's so-called 'religious teachings' were simply a cover for 'disgusting practices', such as enticing teenage girls to his home by advertising a typing job, before proceeding to grope them.[6]

The issue of *The Equinox* in which Boney's parody appeared also contained 'The Temple of Solomon The King IV',[7] unsigned but co-authored by Crowley and Fuller, which treats yoga seriously and compares it to Western science and occultism. In many ways, it is an extension of Fuller's writing on Crowley and yoga in *The Star in the West*. The article, which contains little that would be unfamiliar to anyone conversant with some of the more influential twentieth-century texts on yoga and occultism, concludes with accounts of meditations Crowley allegedly undertook between January and April 1901. The entire piece is heavily indebted to Crowley's former Golden Dawn master Allan Bennett, who the Great Beast had holidayed with in Ceylon in 1901. After that meeting, Bennett decided to go on to Myanmar, where he became a Buddhist monk, while Crowley went to India to study raja yoga before returning to England.

A decade-and-a-half after Boney broke with Crowley, the influence of his former master is readily evident in *Yoga: A Study of the Mystical Philosophy of the Brahmins and Buddhists*. In the book, Fuller cites Hindu yoga and then Buddhism as a means of reaching the highest levels of spiritual understanding, tossing them in alongside Christianity, the whole of Western occultism, the *Qabalah*, and any other esoteric belief he cared to throw into the mix. According to the book's Introduction, yoga philosophy 'has produced the greatest and most influential of masters – Gotama, Christ, Mahomet, whose mastery over the Unknowable has been the driving force of nations'.[8]

The final third of the book is specifically devoted to Buddhism. Given the term 'noble' is understood by some as a synonym for Aryan, it comes as no surprise that Fuller wrote glowingly of 'the noble [or Aryan] eightfold path'. Here, it should be noted that Aryan was originally used simply as a religious, cultural and linguistic identification. The association that Fuller makes with an entirely fictitious racial group – Indo-European for many racists both inside and outside the fascist movement, and more specifically Indo-German for some Nazis – only occurred later.

For Fuller, Buddhism is just another route to ultimate spiritual truth, all esoteric systems being much of a muchness to him. While hierarchical difference mattered for Boney on the so-called racial and social level, he doesn't really distinguish between spiritual systems. In his book, Fuller cites leading theosophist Helena Blavatsky, only to then quote a Hindu source – the *Hatha Yoga Pradipika* – so as to extol its greater exactness![9] Regardless, it appears Blavatsky and Crowley had a greater impact on Fuller's understanding of yoga than the likes of Vivekananda, Mahatma Agamya Paramahamsa, or any of the other Hindu gurus he quotes.

Unlike Blavatsky, Crowley isn't explicitly named in Fuller's book, but it doesn't take a leap of the imagination to work out who 'St. Shamefaced Sex' (a 'potent but middle-class Magician') refers to: 'Even the great science of Yoga has not remained unpolluted by his breath, so that in many cases to avoid shipwreck upon Scylla the Yogi has lost his life in the eddying whirlpools of Charybdis.'[10] Given that Fuller had only broken with Crowley the man, rather than his basic yoga teachings, this put-down should not be taken too seriously.

Likewise, Boney's belief in yoga's equivalence to the *Qabalah* didn't stop him going on to author an anti-Semitic rant in the *Fascist Quarterly* entitled 'The Cancer of Europe',[11] which claimed Jewish people were anti-spiritual materialists who were using magic, money and psychoanalysis to destroy Christian civilisation. In the piece, Fuller deploys the *Zohar* and *Qabalah* to bolster his anti-Semitic bigotry, depicting them as part of the Jewish plot. This was despite his sympathetic use of the same material in his previous book on yoga, and the fact he even included a diagram of The Tree of Life in that work.

The hierarchical caste and spiritual structures of Hinduism – and in particular the authoritarian nature of the relationship between gurus and their students – clearly appealed to full-blown mystical fascists like Fuller. In his book, Fuller writes:

> As the Shiva Sanhita says; '11. Only the knowledge imparted by a Guru is powerful and useful; otherwise it becomes fruitless, weak and very painful. 12. He who attains knowledge by readily pleasing his Guru with every attention, readily obtains success therein. 13. There is not the least doubt that Guru is father, Guru is mother, and Guru is God even: as such he should be served by all, with their thought, word and deed.'[12]

As can be seen, the authoritarian nature of the relationship between gurus and their students – at least as Fuller sees it – mirrors the fascist ideal of the relationship between the Führer and the masses. While Fuller's position as a high-ranking member of the British Union of Fascists and his praise of the Nazis were well known, this didn't stop post-Second World War yogis quoting him in their own books (see below). Fuller's book *Yoga* was still being reissued decades after the military defeat of Nazism. Due to his discipleship with Crowley, his work in this field remains attractive to those of an occult yoga bent, and not just those with explicitly fascist politics.

5

Bengal Lancer and Hitler Aficionado Francis Yeats-Brown

While Fuller was clearly more invested in the metaphysical aspects of yogic practice than in postural techniques, his countryman, fellow British Army officer and Nazi sympathiser Francis Yeats-Brown (1886–1944) emphasised the latter just as much as the former. Yeats-Brown, who was a disciple of Pierre Bernard, briefly found celebrity due to the success of his unreliable yogic memoir, *Bengal Lancer*, published in 1930.[1] In three of his books, Yeats-Brown describes how, having been a Turkish prisoner-of-war, he went on the run by cross-dressing as a German governess. It wasn't his literary squibs, however, that appealed to the Führer, but rather the Hollywood version of Yeats-Brown's fantastical escapades. Hitler reportedly told Yeats-Brown that the Gary Cooper vehicle was one of his favourite films, and had been made compulsory viewing for members of his elite SS. The movie bore about as much resemblance to Yeats-Brown's memoir as the book did to the author's actual life. Like his yoga guru Pierre Bernard, Francis Yeats-Brown was an incorrigible liar.

As is the case for Fuller, historian Kate Imy has done extensive archival research – encompassing manuscripts, diaries and other personal material – into the genealogy of Yeats-Brown's yoga practice. However, while I agree with Imy's conclusion that Yeats-Brown learned the bulk of his yoga at the feet of Pierre Bernard, I diverge in places with her take on this 'fascist yogi'.

While Evelyn Wrench's biography of his cousin Yeats-Brown doesn't mention Pierre Bernard by name, it does have this to say about the period between 1923 and 1925 when the Bengal Lancer's first marriage fell apart and his post-army career stalled: 'Perhaps to regain poise, he studied Yoga at the Yoga centre in Nyack, New York State.'[2] This observation is in accord with the Yeats-Brown material listed as held by the Harry Ransom Center: 'Yoga notebook, handwritten and typed manuscript / notes, approximately 50 pages laid in notebook covers, 1924–1925.' Given Wrench's biography is, alongside the Harry Ransom Center papers, a key source for those looking into Yeats-Brown, it is worth providing a thumbnail assessment of the book.

Wrench's biography was obviously written to serve a number of purposes, and while these shape – and to an extent distort – the work's viewpoint, it is nonetheless considerably more credible than Yeats-Brown's autobiographical writing. Wrench clearly had a deep affection for his cousin, which results in the book brushing over unpleasant details and attempting to portray Yeats-Brown's flaws in the best possible light. Thus, Yeats-Brown's involvement with yoga and fascism are addressed but played down, while his Christian beliefs are emphasised (although not overplayed). In his biography, Wrench is not only defending his family's honour but his personal role as the man who gave the Bengal Lancer his first big break as a journalist, and moreover went on to help him with his career at other times.[3]

Although Wrench writes from a politically and socially conservative perspective, he was firmly opposed to fascism. Moreover, while he clearly wishes to avoid denouncing his cousin's published work as a pack of lies, there are strong indications he doubts the veracity of at least some of Yeats-

Brown's autobiographical material. For instance, Wrench's critical eye is evident in the following passage, which hints that Yeats-Brown's writing about his yogic initiations should not be taken too seriously:

> A few days leave at Christmas enabled him to search for a guru. But Y.B. was ever unsatisfactory as a spiritual pilgrim. He was not the stuff that saints are made of. He lacked the complete concentration essential to the mystic ... One of his friends, Sir Paul Dukes, once referred to him as 'a seeker for a Guru whom he never found'.[4]

Regardless of familial loyalties, as far as basic information about Yeats-Brown's life goes, Wrench provides the most credible published material I've come across. Where facts are disputed, he is the source I would turn to first, unless there is good reason to believe he is wrong on a specific detail. Having drawn attention to Wrench's relative reliability, I now turn to Imy's 'Fascist Yogis', which expands on Yeats-Brown's relationship with Pierre Bernard:

> [Yeats-Brown] filled several notebooks on Bernard's lectures on yoga. Yeats-Brown's subsequent publications and traveling lectures borrowed heavily from Bernard's interpretations, but like Fuller, he chose to not cite his master by name ... [Instead] Yeats-Brown focused on his time in India to validate his claims ... By writing that he had gained control over feverish illness, disobedient bowels, and the desperation of being a prisoner of war, Yeats-Brown used his published works to indicate that yoga provided him with the control over his body that had eluded him as a soldier in the British Empire.

Yeats-Brown's choice to ignore P. A. Bernard and instead argue that his transformative yogic experiences

came from Annie Besant and Indian gurus such as
Bhagawan Sri bears a striking resemblance to Fuller's
unwillingness to refer to Crowley as anything more than
'St. Shamefaced Sex.' Choosing Bhagawan Sri as his official
yogi mirrored twentieth-century ethnographic, orientalist,
and anthropological writers who repudiated the nineteenth-
century European 'experts' in favor of having colonized
people speak. Yet as Fuller's and Yeats-Brown's examples
suggest, this desperation for legitimacy and authenticity
also encouraged fraudulence ... .[5]

Here, Imy uses the term 'fraudulence' to frame the claims of both Yeats-Brown and Fuller as regards their yogic initiations. In the case of Yeats-Brown, non-academic language such as 'total bullshit' seems a more appropriate description of his writing about his mystical mentors (as well as most other matters). Like most other far-right figures attracted to Hinduism, Yeats-Brown seems to have been more inclined to tell people what he believed they wanted to hear, or what made him sound good, than the truth. It is possible to conclude from the books Yeats-Brown published that he did not learn yoga in India before the First World War, but rather at some point after both that conflict and the production of his first autobiographical book, *Caught By The Turks*, published in 1919.[6]

While there is no mention of yoga in *Caught By The Turks*, in later works where Yeats-Brown revisits episodes of his life covered in that book, he adds in the claim he used yoga to survive the ordeal of being imprisoned during the First World War. It can be deduced from this that Yeats-Brown's knowledge of modern postural practice dates from the 1920s. The key event that took place between Yeats-Brown's first book – which was a commercial flop – and *Bengal Lancer* in 1930 appears to be his time studying yoga with Pierre Bernard in Nyack. Having been initiated into the world of yoga by

Bernard, Yeats-Brown clearly made use of what he had learned to craft a far more successful piece of 'non-fiction' than *Caught By The Turks*. Thus, a bestseller was born.

Sometimes described as a military book, *Bengal Lancer* is ultimately a heavily fictionalised account of Yeats-Brown's initiation into yoga in Nyack, New York, despite not a single scene being set at Bernard's Clarkstown Country Club. While *Bengal Lancer* contains reminiscences of military life in India and Europe, including army 'sports' such as polo and hunting wild boar, the meat of the narrative is occult initiation, as evidenced by the titles of the concluding chapters: 'The Festival of the Fish-Eyed Goddess', 'Jaganath, Lord of the World' and 'The Temple of the Undistracted Mind'. At the end of the book is an appendix explaining yoga and its relationship to Christianity for the layperson. Thus, *Bengal Lancer* is part of a long line of bestselling books that draw on Eastern 'spirituality'. It is also a relatively early book about yoga, and certainly an early yoga bestseller. Yeats-Brown's follow-up work, *Lancer At Large*, failed to recapture the success of its predecessor, and is even less convincing in its tall tales of yogic initiation – partly because, rather than being juxtaposed with a life lived as a privileged officer of the British Raj, the yoga is cut into a journalistic fact-finding mission around India.[7]

The Bengal Lancer obviously struggled to find things to write about, and repeatedly re-used material across different books. For example, a seven-page section of *Lancer At Large*, which includes instructions for performing various yoga practices and postures, was recycled in expanded form in *Yoga Explained*.[8] Likewise, the content of *Caught By The Turks* is condensed into a few chapters of *Bengal Lancer*, before being regurgitated at even greater length in *Golden Horn*.[9]

Not all the 'biographical' fictions concerning Yeats-Brown originate with their subject, though. In *Fascist Yogis*, Imy claims: 'Yeats-Brown found in Bernard's club a relatively safe space in which to make personal and professional contacts with American elites and become a minor celebrity by giving airplane demonstrations and telling stories about the war to an adoring audience.'[10] A footnote at the end of this sentence indicates that the author's less-than-reliable source for this assertion is Robert Love's *The Great Oom*. Yeats-Brown was actually in London when Love has him participating in Bernard's flying club. The fact the Bengal Lancer wasn't a pilot and didn't know how to fly a plane render Love and Imy's contentions even more unlikely.[11] Love's biography of Bernard also makes the following dubious claims:

> Major Francis Yeats-Brown, having settled himself in Hollywood to advise on the movie version of *The Lives of a Bengal Lancer*, so impressed Gary Cooper, the film's star, that Coop began experimenting with yoga then and there. Cooper in turn convinced the film's director, Henry Hathaway, to try it, and soon there were others on the set trying out yoga and meditation.[12]

Love provides as his source the story 'Weird Occult Creeds Thrive Among Stars' by Alma Whitaker (*LA Times*, 31 October 1934). Very few people who rigorously research yellow-press 'coverage' of strange happenings in Hollywood accept their content at face value, since they were often no more than entirely fictional PR puffs. According to Wrench's biography, Yeats-Brown was in fact living in Europe while *The Lives of a Bengal Lancer* was being filmed in Hollywood, and there is no mention of his having visited America around this time. The closest date to the Whitaker story specifically referenced in Wrench's book is Sunday, 28 October 1934, when Yeats-Brown had lunch with, among others, Somerset Maugham and Gerald Kelly, and 'drank seven kinds of claret'. While still drunk, he drove down to Tonbridge to see his brother, before returning to London to attend a British Union of Fascists meeting at the Albert Hall, where Oswald Mosley's speech concluded with an 'attack on Jews'.[13]

This was not the only occasion Yeats-Brown went to see Oswald Mosley speak. Wrench writes disapprovingly of a Mosley meeting he attended with his cousin at Olympia in June 1934.[14] While Yeats-Brown received warm receptions from European fascist leaders such as Hitler, Mussolini and Franco, it seems Yeats-Brown's relationship with their British equivalent was more equivocal.[15]

It was also around this time that Yeats-Brown's writing veered towards such unapologetically far-right political diatribes as 1934's *Dogs of War*,[16] a poorly constructed attack on a more successful, pacifist tome called *Cry Havoc!*.[17] The conclusion of the book illustrates the full-blown mystical fascism that runs through both Yeats-Brown's politics and yoga practice:

> We can see only part of the design of nation-building which seems to be God's plan for human progress: but we do discern sometimes how the coulter of war ploughs the world from sleep, and how civilisation had been evolved through the agonies and exultations of conflict. Our own wants and desires are petty beside these cosmic growing pains: physically we die but once, but mystically, through service and sacrifice to our country, we shall live in a body more enduring than our own. Here is an aspect of war which no man has fully fathomed ... Our destiny as a people lies not in subjection to a super-state, but in the dangerous world of the creative will.[18]

It was the Bengal Lancer's insistence on expressing such obnoxious views in political as well as 'spiritual' form that ultimately derailed his journalistic career. Having become the editor of weekly paper *Everyman* at the end of September 1933 – the pinnacle of a journalistic career enabled in large part by family connections – he lost the job in early November of the same year, after overseeing just seven issues. This was because he used his column to espouse the fascist cause, a politically unacceptable line as far as the paper's directors and shareholders were concerned. Yeats-Brown's book sales also withered as their content became more overtly an exposition of fascist ideology. According to Wrench, UK sales declined from a high point of 150,000 (*Bengal Lancer*, 1930) to 30,000 (*Golden Horn*, 1932) and then 5,000 copies (*Dogs of War*, 1934). This was followed by a slight recovery to 'over' 10,000 (*Lancer at Large*, 1936), followed by another dip to 'less than' 4,000 (*Yoga Explained*, 1937). The latter title appears to have had greater success posthumously, having been reprinted in the US, India and Italy after Yeats-Brown's death. Wrench records the first *Bengal Lancer* book as bringing in seven sales for translation rights and the film rights going for $15,000. The only other rights sales he records are for the translation of *Golden Horn* into Italian and Swedish.[19]

Despite being portrayed by Wrench as a failure, *Yoga Explained* clearly sets out Yeats-Brown's vision of modern postural yoga, providing instructions on breathing, meditation, prayer, *chakras*, diet, fasting, enemas and how to improve your memory, as well as descriptions of various postures with accompanying pictures. The illustrations mostly consist of line drawings, but there are also several photographs depicting the scrawny author. Yeats-Brown emphasises meditative breathing over postures, and offers ten 'core' physical exercises (although some of these have variations). The first is lotus, followed up by headstand lotus, apparently also a meditation position. Then there is accomplished pose, which is described as an *asana* for the 'spiritually enlightened' or *siddhasana*. The final meditation pose is thunderbolt, which Yeats-Brown calls 'swastika seat'. There then follows a series of non-meditation poses and exercises, including headstand (with extended legs rather than in lotus position), shoulder stand, plough, seated forward bend, cobra, and a *kriya* consisting of seated body rotations.

Overall, Yeats-Brown's posture practice seems to have consisted chiefly of doing a daily headstand for up to five minutes. In the book, he claims, 'I am supple and healthy for my age; and that, barring accidents, and thanks to being born of healthy parents, as well as to the regular practice of Yoga, I shall probably still be standing on my head in the lotus pose when I am eighty.' He died of heart failure at 58 while being cared for at a nursing home in London.[20]

Yoga Explained contains much padding, long passages of citation, and relentless pseudo-historical nonsense. As a result, Yeats-Brown's propagation of postural practice appears to have had more immediate success in the form of shorter journalistic pieces aimed principally at women. According to the unreliable Robert Love:

> ... a major pivot in the cultural history of yoga in America can be traced to a do-it-yourself article titled 'Yoga for You,' by Major Yeats-Brown, which appeared in the April 1935 issue of *Cosmopolitan* magazine. Yeats-Brown wrote it as an adaptation from his literary contribution to the cause: *Yoga Explained* ... sexy female models illustrated the serpent pose, the lotus seat, the shoulder stand – and the whole package hit the right note at the right time, summoning the do-it-yourself spirit of American women in search of health and beauty in tough times. The *Cosmo* story was further condensed and syndicated, redistributed to hundreds of newspapers under the headline 'Yoga Is Helpful To Mental, Physical Powers.'[21]

If Love's dating of the *Cosmopolitan* article is correct, then it is unlikely it was adapted from *Yoga Explained* as Pierre Bernard's slipshod biographer claims. In *Yoga Explained* – published in 1937 – Yeats-Brown claims on more than one occasion to be 50,[22] which if true would mean he is writing sometime after 15 August 1936. Thus, it is more likely that the widespread success of 'Yoga For You' – assuming Love's details about it are correct – led to the writing of *Yoga Explained*, rather than the other way around

While there is some argument over what can be considered the earliest book-length hatha yoga manual, it is safe to say it wasn't Yeats-Brown's *Yoga Explained*. Pre-dating the Bengal Lancer's book by nearly a decade was *Yogic Physical Culture Or The Secret Of Happiness* by Seetharaman Sundaram (1901–94).[23] In at least some editions of Sundaram's book there is an image of its author in headstand lotus (aka inverted lotus).[24] Sundaram's staging of the pose is rather more impressive than Yeats-Brown's in *Yoga Explained*, in which the scrawny fascist appears to be pulling a pained expression on a rumpled mat. Even so, both this photograph and other aspects of Yeats-Brown's book raise the intriguing question: was *Yoga Explained* influenced by Sundaram's earlier guidebook, or was the latter man somehow influenced by the fascist yogi's guru Pierre Bernard? It is, of course, possible that the two men's influence travelled in both directions.

Returning to Love, he is not the only person to assert that Yeats-Brown had a major impact via the mass media on perceptions of yoga in various parts of the overdeveloped world. Harvey Day, in *Practical Yoga For Women*, takes a rather more negative view of Yeats-Brown's public appeal:

> Unfortunately, pictures of him in inverted postures appeared in the sensational press, which gave the impression that if you took up Yoga it meant standing on your head. That,

very naturally, damped the ardour of the elderly, the obese, the arthritic and those suffering from giddiness, high blood pressure and similar afflictions; in fact, the very people Yoga could help.[25]

That said, it may be some found the racial nationalism that informed Yeats-Brown's understanding of yoga more off-putting than photos of the author standing on his head:

Far from yoga being alien to our racial inheritance, the language in which it was written is our own tongue's grandmother, Sanskrit. Words such as pitr (pater, father), matar, bhratar, duhitar, vidhava (widow) show our family relationship with the first explorers of the Aryan Path ... The blond invaders – Aryans, as it is convenient to call them – were a beef-eating, beer-drinking, horse-loving, pastoral, and poetic folk.[26]

This passage shows Yeats-Brown to be as obsessed with the Aryan origins of yoga as his acquaintance Hamish McLaurin. Both might have looked a little closer to home than the Indus Vallery for the origins of modern yoga, since it clearly has more to do with their guru Pierre Bernard than beef-eating Brahmins.[27] In 1937, the year *Yoga Explained* was published, Yeats-Brown attended Hitler's Nuremberg Rally as part of the British delegation. Wrench uses Nazi interest in *The Lives of a Bengal Lancer* as a way of introducing his cousin's adulatory take on Hitler:

Hitler's appreciation of the film *The Lives of a Bengal Lancer* naturally gratified Y. B. He was present as a correspondent at several of the dramatic events prior to Munich, and had many opportunities of studying the Nazi Leader at close quarters. He writes:

> 'I have met many of the notable figures of the world, but only Gandhi and T. E. Lawrence gave me the sense which Hitler does of inner strength and Franciscan simplicity. All three were ascetics. Complete sexual abstinence would presumably bring the world to an end, if adopted by mankind at large, but practised by rare people like Hitler gives them magnetism and mastery. "Practised" is the wrong word, Hitler is utterly unselfconscious. He lives for his mission, which is to regenerate Germany ... .'[28]

It is telling that Yeats-Brown chose to place the Führer in the same bracket as Mahatma Gandhi, a practitioner of Kriya Yoga. Of course, the former figure's 'Franciscan simplicity' was to have rather more bloodthirsty consequences than the latter's. Nevertheless, Hitler himself had little interest in yoga. Other top Nazis, however, were more open-minded, as the next chapter will show.

As already noted, Yeats-Brown shared his white supremacist views with Hamish McLaurin and both these men had a hand in rolling out Pierre Bernard's brand of embodied spirituality to a global audience. Given that Years-Brown propagated Bernard's exercise system as well as his spiritual grift and garnered far more media coverage for it, he is clearly the key figure here. It was the Bengal Lancer, far more than McLaurin, who blazed a trail for other Oom-connected modern yogis – Paul Dukes and Theos Bernard – to blow credulous minds across the overdeveloped world, as we will see.

6
Jakob Wilhelm Hauer and His Influence on the Architect of the Nazi Holocaust Heinrich Himmler

Several leading Nazis shared Yeats-Brown's obsession with yoga, and in particular his absurd belief that the practice could be traced back to Aryan invaders of the Indus Valley. In fact, chief architect of the Holocaust and Nazi SS leader, Heinrich Himmler, was obsessed by Hinduism as an Aryan religion. Not being a regular reader of the sensationalist UK newspaper the *Daily Mail*, I missed its twisted coverage of this fact in 2012 when it first published the story '"Ve Hav Ways Of Making You Relax": How SS recommended yoga to death camp guards as a good way to de-stress'.[1]

This short piece is a populist – and in places fact-free – reinterpretation of postural yoga teacher and journalist Mathias Tietke's *Yoga im Nationalsozialismus: Konzepte, Kontraste, Konsequenzen*.[2] Tietke details how Himmler was strongly influenced by the views of German Indologist and religious studies writer, Jakob Wilhelm Hauer (1881–1962). Hauer founded the German Faith Movement, which sought to promote a new religion based on Germanic paganism and Nazi ideas. Even with the defeat of the Nazi regime in 1945, Hauer's views continued to influence key yogic practitioners. In a 2006 English-language book that apparently eluded *The*

Mail's researchers, *New Religions and the Nazis,* anthropologist and historian Karla Poewe explains:

> The picture of the world that Hauer sold his followers was one of a fundamental clash (Kampf) between two faith-worlds (Glaubenswelten), the Near-Eastern Semitic and the Indo-German ... The Indo-German faith-world included Hinduism, Buddhism, and a pre-Christian Germanic Faith. Having been a missionary to India ... he personally experienced Hinduism and Buddhism directly and wrote about them professionally. His enchantment with the latter two faiths contributed to his intense, if in his pre-1930 works discreetly expressed, dislike of things and thoughts Jewish. He worked hard behind the scenes to remove Jewish and – what to him amounted to the same thing – Christian scholars from university positions.
>
> By contrast, Hinduism and Buddhism were compatible with National Socialism. Together they blended into an ideological mix that dazzled not only the anthropologists and indologists of the Ahnenerbe ... but pervaded the SS generally from Heinrich Himmler (1900–1945) on down ... .[3]

Poewe stresses Nazi approaches to religion were not uniform, with the likes of Hitler and Goebbels adhering to very different positions on faith compared to figures such as Hauer and Himmler. That said, Hitler was happy to link up with Hindu nationalists in his fight against the British. More crucially, the cod 'Aryan' religious beliefs that pervaded the SS – as well as far-right yoga aficionados – were a key ideological strand that fed into the Final Solution. As Poewe observes:

> Hauer's 1934 publication on the *Bhagavad Gita* lays out systematically the justification for doing the deed that a man is

called to do by fate even if that deed is steeped in guilt ... Hauer calls such a deed innate or hereditary duty (angeborene Pflicht) and there can be little doubt that Himmler saw his destruction of the Jews in that light ... According to Hauer, Krishna taught Arjuna that the 'hereditary duty' has to be done even when it is interlocked with repulsive fate (Schicksal) and with guilt ... In Indo-Aryan times, said Hauer ... this 'innate duty' was equated with the duty that belonged to the caste to which a human being belonged ... For Himmler that caste was the SS.

Poewe then proceeds to quote Peter Padfield:

While there were many paths to perfection, in essence they involved a man doing his caste duty in a disinterested passionless way, dedicating it only to God. And here, perhaps, is the key to the picture of Himmler, by nature a squeamish man, forcing himself silently to watch an extermination at Auschwitz. Performance of duty detached from passion was indeed what he continually sought from his staff at the death camps.[4]

Hauer's interpretation of the *Bhagavad Gita* is, of course, driven by a violent, reactionary political ideology. Nevertheless, it continues to resonate with the way in which yoga, as a form of 'embodied spirituality', is currently taught by a number of yoga organisations in the overdeveloped world. Unfortunately, the effects of Hauer's poisonous 'spiritual' ideology are all-too-evident in the actions of his 'student, later secretary and organizer, Paul Zapp', who:

... received life imprisonment for the murder of at least 13,499 people as leader of the Sonderkommando 11a [an SS and Gestapo mobile killing squad that murdered Jewish people and other targeted groups in the captured territories] and Einsatzgruppe D [an SS paramilitary death squad]. Not surprisingly, he justified his deed [*sic*] in terms of Hauer's and the SD's [*Sicherheitsdienst* or Security Service, i.e., Himmler's SS] religious worldview.[5]

Despite Hauer's close association with various individuals who became convicted war criminals, his reputation after the Second World War was partially salvaged by various disciples and epigones, who went to great lengths to play down their mentor's National Socialist credentials. To this day, Hauer's thinking continues to influence the worlds of yoga and Indology. Perhaps his most visible recent advocate in English-speaking territories is Georg Feuerstein (1947–2012). Although German by birth, Feuerstein lived and worked for much of his adult life in England, the US and Canada, where he devoted himself to yoga, the abusive 'guru' Chogyam Trungpa, and the propagation of ancient Indian sacred texts. Journalist Christopher Locke, in assessing Feuerstein's *The Yoga Tradition: Its History, Literature, Philosophy and Practice*[6] – which he describes as a 'erudite and definitive, New Age Approved, adept and comprehensive study of yoga' – points out that the book contains 'No hint that Herr Doktor Hauer was also a highly enthusiastic Nazi'.[7]

The same criticism can be made of other works by Feuerstein that invoke Hauer, such as his *The Essence of Yoga: A contribution to the Psychohistory of Indian Civilisation*.[8] Feuerstein is popular in yoga circles and according to the biographical blurbs in his books even a patron of the Sport England-recognised British Wheel of Yoga. While Feuerstein's fans – such as yoga teacher and author Richard Rosen – appear to be aware that Hauer's writing helped put their idol on his new age, Indologist life path, they too seem willing to overlook the racial nationalism that underlies it.[9] In failing to address the reactionary, atavistic elements present in yogic discourse and practice, these contemporary practitioners of 'embodied spirituality' effectively turn a blind eye to the fascist origins of their beliefs. Instead, they prioritise the individualistic embrace of 'the spiritual' – that is, a desire for personal realisation. This form of 'spirituality' encourages a callous indifference to not only politics, but the general state of the world.

Running alongside SS ideologist Hauer's ongoing influence on modern postural practice there is a broader and largely mythological discourse about Nazi occultism. In terms of modern yoga, more popular than the *Mail*'s claim that death camp guards used the discipline to de-stress, is the fable that Eva Braun, Hitler's mistress, was a yogini. Phillipa Beck on her Californian postural practice studio Full Circle Yoga website, provides one example of this:

> Berlin's first yoga studio opened in 1937. Books about yoga proliferated, and there were yoga students in 50 German towns and cities. Hitler's wife, Eva Braun, practised yoga, and [postural practice teacher and journalist] Romanelli has dug up a stunning, sunlit photo of her beside a lake in full urdhva dhanurasana (backbend) that could grace the cover of any modern magazine … Hitler was an avid student of yoga and Indian mysticism.[10]

The information in the first two sentences appears to be derived from Tietke's *Yoga im Nationalsozialismus* and may or may not be accurate.[11] The picture of Eva Braun in a back bend that illustrates the essay has been widely reproduced but does it actually show her doing yoga? It is impossible to tell from circulating film and photographs of Braun exercising at Hitler's Berghof mountain retreat in 1942 – including the picture Beck reproduces – whether Hitler's mistress is doing some form of occidental gymnastics or the lightly neo-Hindu seasoned version of such practice known as postural yoga. Evidence from other sources to substantiate assertions Braun is doing yoga seem to be wanting despite the claim being widely repeated in relation to these images. Beck's assertion that 'Hitler was an avid student of yoga' is untrue.

One of the many things that is needed today to help counter the growth of the contemporary far right is a separation of historical fact from fiction. The myth that the Nazis successfully deployed occult forces to ascend to power needs repeated debunking, so that the social and political factors that actually led to their rise become more widely understood. When specifically addressing yoga in relation to this, the starting point should probably be making it clear that Hitler had no interest in the discipline – but as I have tried to show in this chapter, there is a lot more to the subject than just that. Likewise, the uncritical use of a source like the *Daily Mail* for information about Nazi activities by yoga influencer Dave Romanelli, as recorded in my footnotes, is indicative of the credulity of many of those involved in modern postural practice. If yoga influencers are going to take what they read in the *Daily Mail* at face value, they can just as easily fall for fables about their postural practice being a 5,000-year-old tradition that originated in the Indus Valley, or QAnon conspiracy theories, or anti-vax pseudo-science. And some do ... .

7

Mircea Eliade, Julius Evola, Savitri Devi – National Socialism as a Religion and the Yoga of Power

Romanian academic and fiction writer Mircea Eliade (1907–86) is perhaps one of the more visible figures of twentieth-century fascist yoga, despite having attempted after 1945 to hide his previous dalliances with the far right behind a fig-leaf of scholarly respectability. A lot of ink has been spilt in arguments over how close Eliade was to the Iron Guard – a Romanian fascist movement also known as the Legion of the Archangel Michael and the Legionnaire movement – and how much of this was carried over into his later academic work. Either way, his 1935 newspaper review of Julius Evola's *Revolt Against The Modern World* makes it clear that in his youth the prof was fully immersed in far-right racist discourse.[1]

In the review, Eliade references a number of dodgy authors and writings, starting with Alfred Rosenberg's *Myth of the 20th Century* – widely considered to be a key work of National Socialist ideology. Aside from *Mein Kampf*, it is probably the best-known and most widely read book by a high-ranking member of the original Nazi party. Eliade situates Evola – and by implication himself – in a line of far-right, racist thinkers popular with fascists in the 1930s ('Gobineau, Chamberlain, Spengler, Rosenberg'), claiming Evola is 'anti-Christian and anti-political at the same time, as well as opposed to communists and fascists'.

Both Evola and Eliade belong to a clique of revolutionary conservatives – mostly self-styled 'intellectuals'– who positioned themselves to the right of mainstream fascism, which they disdained as too plebeian, too democratic and insufficiently aristocratic for their tastes. The best-known exponent of this ultra-rightist variant of fascist ideology is probably Ernst Jünger, the previously mentioned author of Hitler's favourite book *Storms of Steel* (1920). Also mentioned in Eliade's review is his associate Vasile Lovinescu, who was a disciple of traditionalist writer René Guénon and, under Romanian's wartime fascist regime, would become mayor of his home town of Falticeni.[2]

Although Evola is described in Eliade's review as 'opposed to communists and fascists', during the Second World War he was happy enough to slink around in the shadow of Hitler and Mussolini, and in practice actively supported their fascist regimes in Italy and Germany – even if his religio-political positions were to the right of either leader. Similarly, despite Eliade describing Evola as 'anti-Christian', it was the former who in 1937 introduced the latter to Corneliu Codreanu, leader of the Romanian Christian fascist Iron Guard movement.[3] Evola apparently saw Codreanu as a great spiritual leader, with Eliade claiming he was 'dazzled' by him.

Whether or not Eliade was a fully paid-up member of the Iron Guard is a moot point – it is incontrovertible that he supported and worked for the movement. As historian Mark Sedgwick observes:

> In 1933 Eliade's former teacher and then boss at the university, Nae Ionescu, joined the Legion, in which he was followed by many of his students, including – it would seem – Eliade. There is no record of Eliade's membership, but he

clearly supported the Legion, writing not especially subtle propaganda for it ... The Legionary Movement, according to Eliade, was distinct from all others in being spiritual rather than political. Whereas Communism acted in the name of economics, Fascism in the name of the state, and Nazism in the name of race, the Legionary Movement acted in the name of Christianity. Not that Eliade dismissed race altogether – on at least two occasions he wrote in *Vremea* on the need to purify the Romanian race of Jewish and Hungarian influences ... .[4]

While the traditionalist belief system Eliade learned from Nae Ionescu was later carried over into the former's academic work, he made efforts to veil it given its lack of scholarly rigour, which made it inadmissible within the university system.[5] Not only this, the fascist variant of traditionalism Eliade embraced was deemed ideologically unacceptable after the defeat of the Axis powers. Ultimately, Eliade prioritised his career over his far-right activism and fascist ideology. As a result, there have been heated arguments regarding whether Eliade became apolitical in his later life or in fact remained a fascist. Given that our focus is on Eliade's work on yoga, the core of which was completed during the period in which he was openly a fascist activist and 'intellectual', this debate is not something I will address in any depth. Nevertheless, it is telling that Eliade maintained a correspondence with unrepentant fascist Evola in the post-war period.

Eliade was deeply immersed in far-right activism when he received his PhD in 1933 for a thesis on yoga practices. This was swiftly turned into a book, and proved influential among academics after being translated into French in the mid-1930s. It was revised and expanded after the war, appearing in new form in French in 1954, before being translated into English as *Yoga: Immortality and Freedom* in 1958.[6] Eliade uses his book to describe what he perceives to be the living fossil of yoga and its various practices in granular detail because for him it represents primordial tradition. His work might be understood as an extended description based on Sanskrit religious texts of an unpeeling of the human psyche to decondition it; or rather – at least in Eliade's reworking – to make it accepting of the world as it is and to abandon any striving for things such as social justice.

Many of the categories Eliade conjures up in the book – such as 'India' and 'The West' – appear ridiculously monolithic to the modern eye. Likewise, the idea that for millennia, 'India has been seriously preoccupied with but one great problem – the structure of the human condition' is patently absurd. Most of those on the subcontinent have been more seriously preoccupied with everything from simple survival through to the depredations of colonialism and its plundering ways. Eliade's obsession with separating 'Aryan' from 'pre-Aryan' yogic elements is indicative of his perspectives as a far-right ideologist. Where Eliade invokes 'archaic spirituality', others might see an enthusiasm for class and caste hierarchies.

While Eliade's reputation may have waned within the academy, others still hype him as one of the great twentieth-century writers on religion, and his book on yoga in English translation remains one of the more cited works on the subject. If you understand being mainstream as appealing to thin white women with money to burn, then you can't get more mainstream in the world of modern postural practice than *Yoga Journal* – which in a nine-book long 'Recommended Yogi Reading' list on its website includes Eliade's *Yoga: Immortality and Freedom*.[7] I'm still seeing this work repeatedly recommended to yoga teachers and practitioners with no warning about the fact it was written by someone active in fascist politics at the time it was composed.

FASCIST YOGA

Despite Eliade's academic caution about citing openly traditionalist authors, Julius Evola has five entries in the index of his *Yoga* book; while Nazi Germany's leading academic 'mystic' Jakob Wilhelm Hauer gets 15.[8] Eliade and Evola weren't interested in sport or modern postural practice; for them, yoga merely represents the 'sacred face' of full-blown mystical fascism. What both men wanted was the imposition of hierarchical and feudal religious theocracies across the world.

Compared to Eliade and Hauer, Italian 'super-fascist' Julius Evola (1898–1974) was an obscure figure during the time fascism became an ascendant political ideology. Since the defeat of the Axis powers, however, he has cast an increasingly long shadow as a far-right 'intellectual'.

As a young man, Evola liked to pose as an aristocratic dandy, and had connections to the Futurist and Dadaist movements. Soon enough, however, he gave up poetry and painting – in his view, the avant-garde had become overly commercialised, and therefore was no longer elitist enough for him. At this point, Evola allegedly contemplated suicide, but having rejected this course of action, went on to reinvent himself as a fascist yogi (among other things).

Like Bernard, Evola obscured aspects of his early life, apparently because they were too plebeian for his liking. After being paralysed from the waist down by a shell fragment at the end of the Second World War, Evola mostly spent the rest of his life hanging around his Rome apartment until his death in 1974. He held salons for young fascists, a number of whom would undertake bombings and other acts of terrorism as a way of translating their host's theories into practice.

Today, many members of the alt-right, including Steve Bannon, are proud fans of Evola's books. Among his literary legacy is the excruciatingly turgid *The Yoga of Power: Tantra, Shakti, and the Secret Way*. The book seems to have undergone a number of revisions, apparently starting life as *L'uomo e la potenza* (*Man as Power*, 1926), before assuming its more yoga-explicit main title in 1949. As the subtitle (to the English edition) makes clear, the focus of the book is tantra and Shaktism, which the author was attracted to for the following reasons:

> Although Tantrism is far from rejecting ancient wisdom, it is characterised by a reaction against (1) a hollow and stereotypical ritualism, (2) mere speculation or contemplation, and (3) any asceticism of a unilateral, mortifying, and penitential nature. It opposes to contemplation a path of action [*sic*], of practical realization, and of direct experience ... One among the many Tantric texts remarks rather significantly:
>
> 'It is a womanly thing to establish superiority through convincing arguments; it is a manly thing to conquer the world through one's power. Reasoning, argument, and inference may be the work of other schools (shastras); but the work of the Tantra is to accomplish superhuman and divine events through the force of their own words of power (mantras).'[9]

Having established to his own satisfaction that tantra opposes contemplation by espousing action and practical realisation – thereby embodying a fascist 'warrior ethic' of power – Evola proceeds to give an account of tantra that is both Eurocentric and homogenising, bringing together a diffuse body of religious practices and transforming them into something akin to a single fascist ideology. This mishmash of doctrines would already have been familiar to those acquainted with *Shakti and Shakta: Essays and Addresses on the Shâkta Tantrashâstra* (1918) and *The Serpent Power: The Secrets of Tantric and Shaktic Yoga* (1919), both credited to Arthur Avalon (aka Sir

John Woodroffe). Evola, while acknowledging these sources, manages to rework them into something that is explicitly fascist. Despite the (later) title of his book, Evola does not appear to have actually practiced yoga or tantra himself, and makes clear his information comes pretty much entirely from translations and secondary textual sources:

> I have resolved not to add anything personal or arbitrary: however since my task is not merely to expound but also to interpret esoteric knowledge, which in Tantrism plays a major role, I have been able to substantiate some elements, owing to my ability to read between the lines of the texts, my personal experiences, and the comparisons I have established with parallel teachings found in other esoteric traditions ... .[10]

While those who reject the claims made by tantra's proponents might logically study such rites without practising them, it seems ridiculous for someone like Evola – who claims to have esoteric knowledge and some kind of 'initiation' – to do so. Given that Evola states his belief in the efficacy of tantra, to then assert he can 'read between the lines' of tantric texts while not bothering to engage in the practice himself is as ridiculous as someone who hasn't undergone martial arts training claiming they can read between the lines of karate manuals. Evola concludes *Yoga of Power* by stating:

> I am not even dreaming of proposing Tantrism to the Western world, or of importing it here in the West, so that people may practice it in its original aspects ... Nonetheless, some of Tantrism's fundamental ideas may be considered by those who wish to deal with the problems encountered in our day and age, by assuming avant-garde positions and by attempting new and valid syntheses ...

> Having introduced the reader to a relatively unknown tradition of Hindu spirituality ... having described one of the most interesting forms of yoga, namely kundalini yoga, in the original form, without attempting to adapt or popularise it, I sincerely hope that this present exposition will offer to some readers a few elements for meditation.[11]

Thus, in the course of less than 200 pages, Evola moves from a position in which yoga and tantra stand as examples of primordial 'Aryan' tradition in which contemplation is countered by action and power, to suggesting it might provide fascists such as himself with 'a few elements for meditation' (i.e., contemplation). Here and more generally, despite the ritual invocation of Evola's name as some kind of serious 'thinker' in new age circles and on alt-right websites, his 'ideas' are fatally riddled with contradictions.

When today's alt-right yogis denounce the world we live in as the 'Kali Yuga' — a time of decadence and dissolution — it is a fair bet that this formulation came to them, directly or indirectly, from either Evola or his contemporary Savitri Devi (1905–82). The former uses it interchangeably with the term 'Wolf-Age', something he apparently took from the Norse Edda. Savitri Devi, meanwhile, who appears to be influenced by Evola, was a fascist activist born of an English mother of Italian descent and a French father of Greek descent. Her birth name is Maximiani Portas, but she is better known by her assumed moniker. Like Evola, Devi — who was a devotee of bhakti rather than hatha yoga — was attracted to the 'spiritual' aspects of yoga rather than modern postural practice. She was also a cat lady who disliked taking baths and made a habit of chewing garlic, prompting many to think there was an offensive smell about her unconnected to her odious political views.

Growing out of her obsession with the entirely mythological Aryan origins of the ancient Greeks, Devi developed interests in both Nazism and the Indian caste system. Having become an ardent National Socialist in the late 1920s, Devi travelled to India a few years later in search of 'living pagan Aryanism'. She became a Hindu and in 1940 entered a marriage of convenience with Asit Krishna Mukherji, a local Hindu Nazi. During the war, Devi and her husband engaged in espionage for the Axis powers against the British, acting as go-betweens for their fellow Hindu nationalist Subhas Chandra Bose and the Japanese. Devi is notorious for her view that Hitler was an avatar of the god Vishnu.[12] After the defeat of the Axis powers, she tried to re-found Hitler's National Socialism as a religion.

In her 1958 self-published book, *The Lightning and the Sun*,[13] Devi deploys a Hinduism-infused cyclical view of history — not dissimilar to Evola's reconfiguration of such tropes — involving a steady process of decline from a Golden to a Silver to a Bronze Age, before the final period of 'decadence', called the Kali Yuga (in which we now supposedly live). Devi presents three historical figures as archetypes for understanding history. Firstly, Genghis Khan represents lightning and thus violence, a 'man in time' whose destructive qualities produced historical decay. Secondly, Akhnaton (a pharaoh sometimes also identified as Oedipus or the Biblical Moses) represents the sun, a 'man above time' who used creativity in a bid to transcend historical decay. Finally, Hitler is depicted as a 'man against time' who, by combining both lightning and the sun, will destroy the decayed world and create a new Golden Age. Since Devi claims Kalki (the tenth avatar of Vishnu) will appear to usher in the new Golden Age, this figure stands in for the already dead Hitler (described by Devi as 'he who returns whenever he is needed'; 'the late-born Child of Light', etc.).

Despite being stark raving mad, Devi's ideas didn't disappear without trace. A little later on, Chilean diplomat Miguel Serrano (1917–2009) would proceed to build on the fascist yogic discourse of Evola and Devi and self-publish his own take on Hitler as a supernatural entity and avatar – in three excessively long volumes. Once again, most biographical information circulating about Serrano can be traced back to his own writings and so should be treated with caution, especially the tale of his initiation into an unnamed occult group practising Hitler worship, ritual magic and kundalini yoga in 1942.[14]

While Evola, Devi and Serrano were fully integrated into the relatively small post-Second World War fascist international, what sped their texts into the hands of today's alt-right and the accelerationist neo-Nazi terror cells that operate in the shadows behind it, was their absorption into countercultural fascism. Here the books of Evola and Devi are often literally brandished as totems and talismans, with their treatment as fetish objects often eclipsing their textual content. While Evola and Devi are worshipped as icons of an underground fascist culture, their turgid texts are often more invoked than read. Nonetheless, there are clear parallels between Devi and Serrano's depiction of Hitler as a supernatural entity and the framing of right-wing populist American president Donald Trump as a 'lightworker' in QAnon conspiracy theory.[15] The work of determining how much of this is due to broad mythological structures that lead to the replication of particular features in far-right narratives without any direct knowledge of precursors, and how much to the direct transmission of Devi and Serrano's propaganda via fascist countercultures, is yet to be done.

With regard to those fascist countercultures, as Evola's Italian acolytes engaged in mass murder via bombing campaigns on their home turf during the Years of Lead, his infamy was also spreading in the English-speaking world. Evola himself might not have approved but in the mid-1980s, he became the ideological inspiration for a bunch of

London-based, third-rate post-punk deadbeats, who needed a gimmick to sell their piss-poor music. This traditionalist provided them with a saleable image that propelled them into becoming founding fathers of a global neofolk scene.

Mid-1980s Goth-electronic band Above the Ruins based their name on Evola's book *Man Against The Ruins* (1953, translated into English 2002) and released their sole album *Songs Of The Wolf*, initially only on cassette, circa 1985. In the mid-1980s, they also contributed a track, 'The Killing Zone', to *No Surrender*, a benefit album for the National Front, at the time one of the larger fascist political parties in the UK. This release also featured more conventional Nazi thud, meaning no synthesisers, from Skrewdriver and Brutal Attack. Above the Ruins soon morphed into the long-lasting neofolk group Sol Invictus, whose debut album *Against the Modern World* (1987) was inspired by Evola's book *Revolt Against the Modern World* (1934, translated into English 1995).[16]

Since none of those known to have been involved with Above the Ruins or early Sol Invictus appear to have been able to speak Italian, and the works they were invoking weren't available in English at the time, it is likely they were receiving advice on their image from an 'intellectual' fascist lurking in the background. By 1998, an Evola neofolk tribute compilation album called *Cavalcare La Tigre – Julius Evola: Centenary* had appeared. This featured various European and North American acts from underground rock music scenes associated with Sol Invictus.[17]

Since then, interest in Evola has continued to grow in music genres such as neofolk, power electronics and martial industrial, as a search of record release and music databases will show. These works made a substantial contribution to an explosion of interest in Evola amongst alt-right political groups and neo-Nazi terrorist organisations.

A similar process can be seen in relation to Savitri Devi, starting with the Current 93 album release *Hitler As Kalki* (1993). The title track is based on Devi's belief that Hitler is Kalki, the tenth avatar of Vishnu; it also carries in brackets after it the initials 'SDM', which are generally understood to stand for Savitri Devi Mukherji, the Hitlerite's full married name. The opening and closing tracks both entitled 'Imperium V' seem to be invoking Francis Parker Yockey's notorious fascist/antisemitic book *Imperium: The Philosophy of History and Politics* (1948).[18] The London-based band's name refers to a number of great significance in Aleister Crowley's occult system. It is also possible to buy Current 93 band T-shirts that are advertised as 'Perfect For Beach, Yoga, Exercise, Party Or Hanging Out'.[19]

Underground rock music inspired by and dedicated to Devi and Evola has played a key role in ensuring that an explicitly fascist take on yoga practice continues to circulate among younger white supremacists. That said, taking a cue from the French new right of the 1960s, at least some of those behind the emergence of neofolk in London had a metapolitical strategy whereby they attempted to normalise fascist politics by engaging with mass culture and camouflaging their far-right political views.

This metapolitical strategy was intended to draw potential new recruits into the orbit of the far right without them realising it, so not everyone involved with neofolk necessarily secretly thinks of themselves as a fascist activist. One example of this would be Sean Ragon of the North American neofolk band Cult of Youth, although he has been criticised by anti-fascist commentators for his connections to Death In June[20] (a precursor band to Above the Ruins, Sol Invictus and Current 93) among other things.

Rogan also promotes runic yoga[21] (aka stadha and stadhagaldr), which according to Misty Harker, 'is the use of yoga asanas to invoke the energies of the runes. It was developed by Friedrich Marby and Siegfried Krummer.'[22] While not fascist in origin, runes are also now an integral part of fascist culture and counterculture. Marby and Krummer's early twentieth-century rune gymnastics and rune dancing appear to have been transformed in the 1980s into rune yoga, tantra, mantras and mudras, by right-leaning US 'Germanic' occultist Stephen Flowers aka Edred Thorsson.[23] Runic yoga has evolved from there, with the likes of Misty Harker who writes about it online, also listing a yoga teacher qualification on her blog. As I've seen it performed, it looks like a postural practice flow sequence in which the limbs are used to mimic the shapes of runes — if I'd first come across it by chance being performed in a doom-metal yoga class, it wouldn't have given me pause for thought.

Serrano proved more popular in genres other than neofolk, including the openly neo-Nazi national socialist black metal scene.[24]

PART III

Downward Dog: Occult Madness and Yogic Televangelism (Modern Postural Practice in the Post-War Era)

Fascist Yoga

After the Second World War, openly fascist yoga unsurprisingly became a minority pursuit and – aside from those who saw themselves as hardcore disciples of the likes of Pound, Evola and Devi – most involved with yoga were circumspect about far-right ideological influences. Of course, that is not to say the influence of white supremacists such as Pierre Barnard and his ilk did not endure in the following decades. As we will see, much of the hucksterism and cod-philosophy that Bernard helped cultivate was on full display among many of those practising (and selling) postural practice in the years after his death. Drawing on the faux-oriental wisdom and fabricated historical timeline that had been elaborated in the pre-war years, the yoga scene's continuing irrationalism left the door open for the return of its repressed far-right racist elements once the horrors of Nazism began to fade from living memory.

Today, much of what passes for the history of modern postural practice is a product of cognitive bias. Images of the Indian subcontinent and ascetics loom large in the popular imagination when it comes to yoga. While Pierre Bernard is undoubtedly a key figure in the spread of modern yoga, both directly and through his disciples, he was for a long time largely forgotten. Bernard's revival as a figure of historical interest came at the price of journalists forging an unproven, possibly entirely fictitious link between him and the Indian subcontinent via the ghostly guru figure of Sylvais Hamati. The same journalists also chose to ignore the immersion of Bernard's immediate circle in Aryanism.

While it is perhaps unsurprising that in the aftermath of Hitler's fall the yoga world did not want to tie its history to the likes of Francis Yeats-Brown, Bernard's other once-prominent British disciple Paul Dukes hasn't been much talked about in recent years either, despite being less politically problematic. As the following chapters will show, Pierre Bernard and his circle remained a major force in modern postural practice into the second half of the twentieth century. Bernard's influence is most immediately apparent through his nephew Theos Bernard, as well as the two British figures just mentioned.

In *Yoga in Britain: Stretching Spirituality and Educating Yogis*, Suzanne Newcombe asserts that 'It is only by considering yoga in precise locations that statements about yoga's significance and effects can have any meaning.'[1] Much of what the chapters thus far have examined locates yoga in the overlapping worlds of transatlantic fascist ideology, esoteric belief and con-artistry. Moving into the post-Second World War period, the emphasis now falls much more on the latter two elements. At the same time, given the many personal ties between key figures in the yoga world from this era, it makes most sense to adopt a transatlantic perspective in attempting to unpick the development of postural practice – and its associated orientalist spiritual ideology – as opposed to simply focusing on either the British Isles or North America.

For example, given his extensive connections in a variety of reactionary milieus, it is difficult to make sense of someone like Francis Yeats-Brown without looking at both fascist networking across Europe in the inter-war period *and* the scene around Pierre Bernard in Nyack, New York. Although part of Yeats-Brown's life was famously played out in India, this is of far less significance when it comes to his yoga practice than the US and European contexts. Since modern postural practice is so clearly a product of cultural hybridity, Newcombe could just as well have written that it is only by considering yoga as having developed across *multiple* geographical locations that statements about its significance and effects can have any meaning.

Moving on, Indra Devi, described as 'the woman who brought yoga to the West', has in recent years enjoyed a historical revival. Her influence on modern postural practice is, again, felt both directly and through associates such as Michael Volin. The latter is now largely forgotten, but according to Devi's biographer was once known as 'the man who brought yoga to Australia'.[2] Devi has probably fared better in terms of renown than Volin in part because — as we will see in Chapter 9 — it looks like she learned her yoga in India, while her associate claimed to have received his basic training in China.[3] Devi had books on yoga published before Volin — although the latter was more prolific and seems to have been as widely translated — but I only cover the former, who has a much higher contemporary reputation and more ongoing influence. That said, those reviving Devi as a figure of interest within the history of yoga tend to gloss over her snobbish attitudes and demented occult beliefs.

The post-war years also saw an intensifying trend towards hucksterism, with the money-making opportunities offered by the West's growing interest in yogic exercise exploited to the max by personalities such as James Lee-Richardson (aka Desmond Dunne), Richard Hittleman and the 'Einstein of the Occult', Frank Randolph Young. These men don't seem to have had any direct connection to the Indian subcontinent, although the Panamanian-born Young claimed to be a descendant of Indian yogis. While these figures have been largely ignored by the majority of contemporary yoga historians, back in the second half of the twentieth century their yogic texts were consumed by the bucketload and they played a huge role in the growth of modern postural practice. Hittleman seems to have had greater ongoing audience reach than any other yogi in the 1960s and 1970s through his postural exercise TV shows. He was the only yoga practitioner I'd heard of when I was a child. Unlike Hittleman, the likes of Lilias Folan weren't as quick to get their media careers kick-started and their postural practice TV shows weren't broadcast in Europe.

While these modern yogis tended to drop overt fascism from their arsenal of bonkers beliefs, Young in particular was not far removed from such extremism, and many others did everything in their power to propagate either pseudo-scientific occult superstitions or faith-based anti-scientific worldviews. However, it was the rise of the anti-masking and anti-vax pastel QAnon movement that prompted mainstream media commentators to really sit up and take notice that the yoga world was riddled with far-right nutjobs. This was the QAnon conspiracy with a feminine touch and pastel wellness aesthetics, in which the claim that Donald Trump was going to save the world from a fictitious cabal of Satanic child-abusing cannibals was put across with a smile rather than a snarl. One of the most visible modern postural practice QAnon cheerleaders in an era of life-saving lockdowns, sensible social distancing and necessary mask mandates was social media influencer Krystal Tini.[4] Tini had already come to the attention of the wellness world through her company My Soul Mat, which sold overpriced and ugly yoga accessories. Tini said of herself in 2019:

> I've struggled with depression, anxiety, and even [*sic*] diagnosed with borderline personality disorder recently. All of these factors led me to the importance of affirmations and utilizing them in my life. If I just had positive statements to look at in [yoga] class with gorgeous images and colors staring back at me, I would focus on those mantras. And it worked.[5]

The twentieth-century yogis covered below kept the irrational world of wellness fertile for the far right through the Cold War years, spreading deluded beliefs that pastel QAnon boosters such as Tini treated as a pick-and-mix from which to collage together their hate-mongering social media posts.

8
Paul Dukes, Francis Yeats-Brown (Again) and Theos Bernard, Spreading the Great Oom's Gospel in the Post-war Years

One key beneficiary of Pierre Bernard's tendency to fish for yoga disciples among heiresses was the previously mentioned British musician, author and spy Paul Dukes (1889–1967). A clergyman's son, Dukes married Margaret Rutherfurd – whom, as previously mentioned, Bernard cultivated – in 1922. Although Dukes joined Bernard's Nyack commune before his friend Francis Yeats-Brown, he wasn't as fast off the mark in promoting modern postural practice to the broader public. That said, Dukes is, or at least was, best known to the wider public for writing and talking about his anti-Bolshevik antics in Russia during the early part of the twentieth century. While Dukes may have been a reactionary, he was not a fascist. Nevertheless, he did have a key role to play in propagating Barnard's vision of yoga, and thus the modern Western postural yoga we see today.

Many believe that the – sadly unpreserved – short series of programmes about yoga Dukes made for the BBC in 1948/9 marks the first time the subject was addressed on television. The photographic section of Dukes' book, *The Unending*

Quest: Autobiographical Sketches, contains three pictures taken from the filming of the shows.[1] In all three, Dukes is seen practicing yoga with the assistance of three scantily clad women referred to as coming from the London-based Legat School of Russian Ballet. In the first picture, a woman stands on Dukes' stomach while another holds her arm, presumably to assist with balance. The second shows Dukes with a stool beneath his glutes, while one dancer places her hands on his back and forehead, and another holds a hand above his feet, almost as if she is trying to levitate him. Finally, the third shows Dukes and two dancers in basket headstands, with a caption that states: 'Final tableau of a television demonstration: headstands on a revolving dais.' Supposedly, the BBC were less than happy with Dukes' salacious behaviour and on-air promotion of the Legat School.[2]

Overall, the impression given by the photographs is of yoga being presented to a television audience as spectacle, akin to the feel of circus and carnival attractions. In doing so, it recalls how Pierre Bernard emerged into public view as something of a sideshow act. When narrating in *The Unending Quest* how he came to be introduced to Bernard and yoga more generally in the early 1920s, Dukes places great emphasis on the importance of headstand. First, he writes of talking about yoga to acquaintances in Nyack, most of whom respond with horror before proceeding to tell him about Bernard's Clarkstown Country Club. As Dukes reports it: '"They stand on their heads!" said another oleaginous female, as if this feat were especially obscene. "They stand on their heads men and women together!"'[3]

Intrigued, Dukes visits Bernard's yoga centre, where – prior to meeting the Great Oom – he encounters an English instructor called Corbin who explains the significance of the headstand. According to Corbin, since blood in the stomachs of quadrupeds flows horizontally, they aren't in the same danger of their internal organs suffering a prolapse compared to humans, who are faced with gravity dragging their stomach blood downwards. Therefore, Bernard and his instructors get their students to stand on their heads in order to allow gravity to pull the blood in the opposite direction. Corbin also claims a headstand 'gives the brain a blood bath at the same time – you know the brain requires more blood than the rest of the body. To stand on the head for a few moments is a sort of physiological cocktail whenever you feel fagged.'[4]

Since Bernard published little, we must rely on the work of his students to provide us with a rough guide to his practice. From this, we can deduce headstands were an important part of Bernard's system. For example, a stress on inversions is also evident in Francis Yeats-Brown's *Yoga Explained*, which, in recommending ten *asanas* for home practice, states: 'I do them all occasionally, except the cobra pose, but I do none of them regularly except the head-stand.'[5] The book also features a photograph of Yeats-Brown doing a tripod headstand lotus,[6] along with a series of drawings depicting how to achieve a basket headstand.[7] Similar instructions on how to do headstands can be found in two books by Paul Dukes: *Yoga For The Western World* and *The Yoga Of Health, Youth and Joy*.[8] As is the case for many older yoga manuals, *asanas* such as downward dog and flow sequences such as sun salutations are absent, with yoga presented more as a series of static poses.

Meanwhile, Pierre Bernard's nephew Theos Bernard (1908–47), who published a relatively early Western yoga manual in 1944 entitled *Hatha Yoga: The Report of a Personal Experience*, was another important figure in ensuring his uncle's teachings endured after his death. Short of funds in his early life, Theos married money in the form of heiress Viola Wertheim, one of his uncle's followers. The marriage eventually failed but before it did so, Theos managed to extract sufficient funds to study and travel to India. After spinning a series of tall tales about yoga and Tibet, Theos scored some sensational press coverage. In 1947, Theos disappeared in the Punjab, assumed to have become one of innumerable victims of the inter-communal violence associated with the Partition of India. His body was never found.

Theos appears to have been taught yoga by his father Glen Bernard in the early 1930s. However, taking a leaf out of his uncle's book, he fictionalised the process to make others think he had learned the practice under a guru from the Indian subcontinent.[9] As scholar Paul G. Hackett observes: 'numerous primary source materials have become available that shed light on [Theos] Bernard's actual activities and the man behind the self-constructed mythology, revealing much of the content of his "autobiographies" to be fictitious or misrepresentative of the actual events in his life.'[10]

In the mid-1930s, Theos Bernard spent time with his uncle on the East Coast, meaning it is likely his practice from this point on was directly influenced by Pierre Bernard.[11] At this time, it seems he had already learnt hatha yoga from his father.[12] Therefore, it is worth asking who exactly taught Theos' father, Glen Bernard, yoga?

As described previously, journalist Robert Love claims Pierre Bernard learned yoga from a shadowy – and possibly non-existent – guru named Sylvais Hamati. So it is unsurprising that Love answers the above question by pointing in the same direction: 'Glen was ... handed over to Hamati, who undertook the task of training another member of the Bernard clan.'[13] Love attributes the information to 'Glen A Bernard, letter from Theos Bernard Collection, University of California at Berkeley; cited in Paul Gerald Hackett, 'Barbarian Lands: Theos Bernard, Tibet and American Religious Life' (doctoral thesis, Columbia University, 2008)'.[14] In his book based on the above-mentioned doctoral thesis, however, Hackett says: 'Glen states that he left home at the age of nineteen in 1903, at which point he appears to have joined his brother, Pierre, who introduced him to yoga and his guru Hamati ... For a more detailed chronology of these events and the life of Glen's older brother, see Love, *The Great Oom*.'[15] In other words, we are going around in circles: Love refers us to Hackett as a source and Hackett then steers the reader back to Love for more detail on the matter. Put simply, there is no independent source (at least that I'm aware of) that reliably establishes whether either of the Bernard brothers learned yoga from a guru called Hamati. In light of Hackett's comment that Glen claims to have been introduced to yoga by his brother, it seems more likely that Pierre Bernard himself was Glen's first – and possibly only – yoga teacher.

Either way, given Glen was – at least according to Hackett – involved in his brother's dubious yogic business operations, his statements on such matters should also be treated with caution. Hackett, though, takes at least some of Glen Bernard's unsubstantiated assertions at face value: 'Glen also claimed to have met an Indian yoga teacher as a teenager and *in his case, it was true* [emphasis added]. Like the vast majority of events recounted in *Heaven Lies Within Us*, this "meeting" between a teenage boy and an India guru refers to Glen Bernard and, presumably, Sylvais Hamati.'[16] Theos Bernard's book *Heaven Lies Within Us* has been widely debunked, including by Hackett himself, who assumes that Theos dishonestly appropriated the life story of his father. One possible conclusion is that Theos resorted to repeating tall tales spun by his father to promote family business interests at the start of the twentieth century, when his father and uncle were apparently engaged in offering the public dubious medical cures.

Here, it is worth noting that Hackett backs up his supposition about Hamati by way of a reference to the unreliable Love. Regardless of whether the real facts about the origins of the Bernard family's postural practice can ever be disentangled, Theos Bernard's *asana* teaching has clear similarities to that of his uncle's disciple Yeats-Brown, who also fabricated an Indian source for his practice.

In terms of the impact of Theos' book *Hatha Yoga*, Suzanne Newcombe is probably over-egging things with her claim that the wealthy Aleister Crowley-disciple and part-time British book editor:

> ... Gerald J. Yorke was personally involved with introducing the first three major circulating books on 'hatha yoga' to the British public; Bernard's *Hatha Yoga* (1944), Yesudian and Haich's *Yoga and Health* (1953), as well as *Light on Yoga* (1965). Both *Hatha Yoga* and *Yoga and Health* were considered to be very successful in profit margins and sales figures.[17]

Rather, like Yeats-Brown, Theos Bernard probably made the most impact through the newspaper and magazine coverage he garnered.

9
Indra Devi and Her Editors at Prentice Hall

Indra Devi (1899–2002) may not be a household name but she enjoys a certain fame in the world of modern postural practice, due in part to the fact she taught a gentle yoga practice to a number of 1950s Hollywood icons, including Greta Garbo, Eva Gabor and Gloria Swanson. Her reflected celebrity as a personal trainer to the stars provided her with a platform from which to spread dubious claims about yoga. Devi has been variously described as 'the first lady of yoga', 'the woman who brought yoga to the West' and the teacher who 'planted the seeds for the yoga boom of the 1990s'.[1] Comparing the biographical information in Devi's books with other sources – including the biography written by Michelle Goldberg – the distinct possibility emerges that these various accounts all originate from information supplied by Devi herself. As such, much of what is repeatedly claimed about Devi's life – especially before her arrival in the US – should be treated with caution.

Born Eugenie Peterson in Riga, Latvia, to a Russian mother and Swedish father, Devi was later displaced by the Russian Revolution. Devi's father was supposedly a White Army officer who went missing in action while fighting the Bolsheviks. Having lost their family fortune during the civil war, Devi and her mother floated around Europe for something approaching a decade.

Downward Dog: Occult Madness and Yogic Televangelism

An encounter as a teenager with the book *Fourteen Lessons in Yogi Philosophy and Oriental Occultism* by fake guru Yogi Ramacharaka – in reality, William Walker Atkinson – sparked Devi's interest in India. Adult encounters with theosophy later cemented her obsession. Having moved to the Indian subcontinent, she became interested in postural yoga and used her personal connections to become a student of Tirumalai Krishnamacharya, a man with an impressively and demonstrably fake guru lineage. When her husband was posted to China, Krishnamacharya told her to go and teach yoga there.

Following the death of her spouse, Devi wound up in Los Angeles, where from the late 1940s she continued to push Krishnamacharya's Hindu-cloaked version of European gymnastics. In the early 1950s, publisher Prentice Hall contracted Devi to write *Forever Young, Forever Healthy*, with 'assistance' from Sidney Field.[2] Devi suggests the decisive factor in landing her US publishing deal was the existence of her first book, *Yoga: The Technique of Health and Happiness*, which had been published in India: 'It was my Indian volume that gave Prentice Hall the idea of publishing one in this country.'[3] Those with a more cynical bent may argue that it was Devi's celebrity students more than her ability to write that attracted the publisher.

Before delving into Devi's publications, it is worth noting what writer Elizabeth Kadetsky is quoted as saying about Devi's teacher in *The Path Of Modern Yoga*:

> Krishnamacharya's story about discovering a hermit in the caves of Tibet in the deep Himalaya, circa 1915, and imbibing the wisdom of yoga as preserved in the caves since the tenth century, does not really stand up to investigation ... the whole story is laced with mystical details. So maybe Krishnamacharya never went to Tibet.[4]

Going further, American Indologist David Gordon White deconstructs the various contradictory biographical claims made by and about Krishnamacharya, revealing them to be at best implausible and in all likelihood impossible.[5] Once again, we are faced with the familiar story of an individual claiming to have been initiated into supposedly ancient yogic practices by a teacher whose very existence may be questioned.

In *The Path of Modern Yoga*, Elliott Goldberg details how, in the mid-twentieth century, occidental practices were adapted by yoga teachers on the Indian subcontinent, whose belligerent nationalism then led them to claim their adaptations of Western physical culture were in fact native traditions:

> ... yogis in early 20th-century India refused to acknowledge that their transmutation of yoga into an exercise system for fitness and health was inspired by Sandow, Müller, Macfadden, and other leaders of the physical culture movement in Europe and America. Instead they dismissed Western exercise systems as recent, inferior versions of centuries-old, indigenous Indian practice.[6]

Fakery and fraud among those given to passing off modernist innovations as 'ancient knowledge' — embodied or not — is nothing new. That said, there is something peculiarly American about the hucksterism of Devi's book *Forever Young, Forever Healthy*, which incorporates sham case studies about the benefits of yoga throughout. One particularly egregious example is the following:

> Let me tell you, for example, of a sixteen-year-old girl, Eva P. Her physical and mental development was retarded due to meningitis at the age of eight. She remained illiterate because of her feeble mind, and could not even do simple domestic work ... After three months of Yoga exer-

cises she began to change from a sloppy, morose and timid creature into a pleasant and tidy girl, smiling and communicative ... Fifteen months later she became an apprentice in a hair dressing shop. No one could recognize in the comely looking girl the unfortunate little imbecile she had been not so long before.[7]

Unsubstantiated case studies of this type will be all too familiar to readers of old books on new age and occult themes issued by Prentice Hall. I return to this publisher and its Parker imprint in the chapters dedicated to Richard Hittleman and Frank Rudolph Young. While some of the authors responsible for Prentice Hall titles may have been deluded enough to believe what they wrote, the attitude of their editors was utterly cynical. In 2014, *This American Life* broadcast a radio programme about Prentice Hall editor Joseph Schaumberger penning a spurious occult self-help manual after seeing how much more money those whose books he facilitated made from their works than he did. The resultant work, *Ultra-Psychonics*, was credited to Walter Delaney, a pen name taken from a make of flush toilet. Although Schaumberger died before the radio show was recorded, his daughter Barbara was interviewed and made clear her father wrote the book as a self-enrichment exercise. He and his family considered it ridiculous that some readers actually believed in the pseudo-scientific occult techniques he described.[8]

Returning to Devi's first book for Prentice Hall, *Forever Young*, the initial 128 pages are taken up with a (presumably) ghost-written 'autobiography', followed by chapters on topics such as breathing, relaxation, diet, endocrine glands, or using yoga to cure common ailments. It is only the final 40 pages of the book that are given over to the usual illustrated yoga exercises, including lotus headstand. According to Devi (or at least her ghostwriter and/or editors), standing on your head is a great way to cure 'headaches, nervousness, sleeplessness, indigestion, constipation, asthma, congested throat, liver, spleen, eye and nose troubles (initial stages), seminal weakness, ovary and uterus troubles'.[9]

As we have seen, Devi is far from alone in making spurious claims about the benefits of headstand practice. Sometimes the fraudulent medical assertions made about the benefits of this particular *asana* are combined with other forms of quackery. For example, in a 1966 address to the Congress of the British Society of Dowsers, J. Armshaw claimed headstands improve dowsing ability – that is, locating ground water or other objects and materials through divination: 'The posture called the "Pole" ... consists of standing on one's head ... Ten minutes of this posture each day can work wonders so far as dowsing sensitivity is concerned.'[10] Such pseudo-scientific nonsense is perfectly of a piece with Devi's occult beliefs, which we will return to below.

Devi's follow-up to *Forever Young* was *Yoga For Americans*[11] – published as *Yoga For You* in the UK[12] – which also features spurious case studies, although the bulk of them are presented as letters to the author and tucked away in an appendix. How many of these letters are genuine is a moot point.

The book's exercises are introduced earlier than in Devi's previous effort, although not until the author has explained the reason she felt compelled to pen another yoga tome:

> The desire to give a clearer understanding of Yoga and the possibility of studying its health methods at home were what actually spurred me on in writing this book, especially after I had learned of the shocking state of the national health in the United States, where physical and mental illness statistics are ever increasing, and the number of alcoholics, narcotic addicts, delinquents and criminals is growing by leaps and bounds.[13]

Following this rant, which minus the yoga sounds more like a speech by a die-hard political conservative, we move on to the exercises. Again, the emphasis is on headstands. Alongside the *asanas* – including a number of potentially risky backbends – there is much about diet. The book also has a week-by-week exercise plan, with the first week providing additional information on honey and coffee enemas. According to Devi, the latter can 'arrest the beginning of a cold or stop a toxic headache', although she cautions: 'It is best *not* to take a coffee enema late in the evening, however, to avoid being kept awake at night.'[14] The poses are illustrated by everyone from Hollywood A-lister Gloria Swanson to an old woman described as Devi's 77-year-old mother. There are no illustrations demonstrating how to perform the enemas.

In general, the book adheres to the established yoga manual formula: explaining how to do a pose before expanding on its supposed health benefits. Elliott Goldberg has argued that particular therapeutic values should not be ascribed to individual *asanas*, as is the case in Devi book's and many yoga titles. Tracing this practice back to Jagannath Ganesh Gune, aka Swami Kuvalayananda (1883–1966), Goldberg observes of Kuvalayananda's self-proclaimed 'scientific' research:

> … these case studies are so flimsy that they don't even lend themselves to generating or testing hypotheses. As evidence for *Sarvangasana* (shoulder stand) treatment curing leprosy, testicular degeneration, epilepsy, poor venous circulation, premature ejaculation, and erectile dysfunction, they're more like a collection of old wives' tales than case studies.[15]

Returning to Devi, spurious medical claims and fake testimonials are not the only means she employs in padding out *Yoga For Americans* to book length. Each section, having set out a week's worth of poses and breathing exercises, concludes with passages given over to topics only vaguely related to yoga, many of which reveal the influence of theosophy and other occult interests. For example:

> Alcohol is avoided by the yogis because it lowers the vibrations of their astral body, whereas the purpose of Yoga is to heighten these vibrations ... Smoking is also supposed to coarsen and make breakable the astral web, which in a developed individual should be thin and strong enough to protect him from the lower influences.[16]

Fifty pages on, there is a section entitled 'On The Kundalini Power', which having spun the usual occult fictions about *chakras*, concludes with a quote from notorious fascist yogi and Western occultist Major General J. F. C. Fuller: 'The yoga philosophy has been the solace of millions for many centuries, not only in India but throughout the world. This philosophy has produced the greatest and most influential masters, Gautama, Christ, Mohammed, whose mastery over the Unknowable has been the driving force of nations.'[17]

As this reverent use of Fuller's words of wisdom implies, while fascism as a political philosophy may have been utterly discredited in the post-war world, that didn't stop Devi – among many others – taking advantage of the pre-war fascists' cod-Hindu philosophy and false claims about yoga's history in promoting their practice. On Devi's part, the apparent contempt for the masses that seeps through her writing echoes the rhetoric of those on the far right who vilify great swathes of the population while looking to 'superior' figures to act as the driving force of nations:

> You can also use the Recharging breath for protecting yourself against the disturbing influences of gross or depressing vibrations ... In India one often does that when

traveling a long distance by train with people whose vibrations might be of a low or an evil order. A friend of mine, a well-known artist in California, found himself doing it, too, when using subway and buses in New York, as he was so sensitive to alien vibrations that they would make him feel almost sick.[18]

This, then, is the deluded, snobbish mindset of an occult crank revered by many as a towering pioneer of modern yoga in the West.

10
Harvey Day, a Hack Who Found Success with Books on Yoga

British author Harvey Day (1903–93) included sun salutations in a yoga manual a decade before Indra Devi got around to putting them in one of her books.[1] Once a popular writer of influential yoga and occult books, he is now largely forgotten. Nevertheless, he remains pertinent to the story of post-war postural practice for a number of reasons. Firstly, despite obviously detesting Nazism, he still felt compelled to invoke the entirely fake Aryan origin story of yoga propagated by the white supremacists described in the earlier parts of the book. Secondly, his books on yoga give a representative impression of the types of cod-spiritual nonsense that was prevalent at the time. Thirdly, he had a propensity to repeat other people's tall tales, making him in effect a forerunner to more recent popular writing on modern yoga that unquestioningly regurgitates whatever nonsense the author can lay their hands on (yes, Robert Love, I'm looking at you). And fourthly, the bibliography of titles he draws on in expounding on yogic practice offers a useful window into the publishing landscape at the time, and more specifically who else was prominent in spreading the distorted ideas formulated by Bernard and the fascists who followed in his wake.

The details of Day's life are somewhat sketchy. The British Library catalogue provides his full name as being Harry

Harvey Day, although he used a number of pseudonyms, including P. E. Norris. According to his author biography on the dust jacket of *The Occult Illustrated Dictionary*:

> Harvey Day was born in Rajbari, Bengal [now Bangladesh], where he developed an interest in yoga and the occult. After training for some time as an electrical and mechanical engineer with the Eastern Bengal Railway, he went to Britain to gain further qualifications in this field, but instead became a freelance journalist.[2]

In his book, *You, Too, Can Write For Money*, Day explains that he came to earn a living from journalism by researching what editors wanted while writing about what he knew but others didn't. Among other things, he addressed daily life on the Indian subcontinent and sports from a colonial perspective. Alongside this, Day claims to have read extensively on health and diet, allowing him to churn out articles on related subjects. It was these principles that drove his writing on yoga:

> I studied yoga and had met yogis in India, and after the war realised that a really simple work on the subject was badly needed. It was this that led me to write *About Yoga*, which sold enough copies for the publisher to invite me to follow it with *The Study and Practice of Yoga*.[3]

Day managed to keep getting his books published from 1951 until 1987. What isn't evident from the autobiographical sketch he provides in *You, Too, Can Write For Money* is his deep interest in the occult, for which his books on yoga provided an outlet. Turning to his 1951 work *About Yoga: The Complete Philosophy*, Day warns readers at the outset that while it is impossible to become 'a compleat yogi' in Britain, some useful knowledge of the subject is possible.[4] He proceeds to claim that he benefits from 'the constant practise of certain mental, physical and spiritual exercises adapted to suit my western way of living',[5] before describing himself as a sickly child whose interest in diet and physical culture – including yoga – cured him of health problems:

> I was born in the malarial swaps of India ... For the first fifteen years hardly a week went by without a bout of malaria, ague or dengue. If I rose free of fever and lay down the same night without a rise in temperature, I felt that the gods had worked a minor miracle.[6]

The trope of the sickly child cured by a miracle fitness regime is a staple of the genre. In *About Yoga*, Day asserts sport and plain food at school rectified his ill-health. He also reports that his teachers recommended deep breathing and exercises sometimes based on yoga. Day also read several books by American proponent of physical culture Bernarr McFadden and claims a number of the exercises contained within them were derived from yoga – although it would probably be more accurate to reverse this direction of travel.[7] Day also says he met yogis and witnessed them perform miracles: 'From my very earliest days I never doubted that yogis and fakirs possessed powers that ordinary mortals did not.'[8]

Day says he picked up his yoga here and there, never applying himself to any serious study of the subject: 'My early excursions into yoga were haphazard. I did not sit at the feet of a *guru* (teacher) but picked up scraps from various adepts as I went along.'[9] In this respect, the words Day devotes to Alexander Cannon (1896–1963) – the so-called 'Yorkshire Yogi' who had a lucrative practice in hypnotherapy and alternative medicine – are telling.[10] In *About Yoga* and his later *Yoga Illustrated Dictionary* and *Occult Illustrated Dictionary*,[11] Day uncritically accepts Cannon's claims to have successfully levitated. Funnily enough, one of the tales *not* recounted by Day in this regard concerns an attempted levitation of a young woman by Cannon in May 1934 at the Mayfair Hotel in London:

> Witnesses said the girl obviously seemed like she was in a trance but the experiment failed. She was not levitated. Dr. Cannon attributed his failure on the weight of the girl's clothes claiming 'that the experiment would have succeeded had it been feasible to strip the girl in the main lounge of the hotel'.[12]

Nevertheless, Day insists in *About Yoga* that 'There are many physical and mental benefits to be gained by the regular and meticulous practice of Hatha yoga, and in the very advanced stages such apparent miracles as levitation can be achieved.'[13] Having recounted a selection of yoga 'miracles', he moves on to yet another well-established trope of mid-century yoga books – the Aryan origins of the practice:

> Many scholars and archaeologists believe that the earliest civilisation existed somewhere in Mesopotamia, a civilisation earlier even than that of China, and that these people spread gradually to Central Asia. It was their ancestors, known as Aryans, who invaded India about 3,000 B.C. and imposed their culture on the aborigines.[14]

Despite the above appearing to echo the narrative provided by the pre-war fascist practitioners of yoga, and while Day mentions Francis Yeats-Brown in passing and includes his work in the book's short one-page bibliography, he clearly detests Nazism and at times expresses explicitly anti-racist views.[15] Even so, the supposed Aryan origins of yoga are so deeply ingrained in his understanding of the practice that he is compelled to comment: 'In primitive communities physical fitness is a prime asset, for only by physical fitness and prowess does one eat and exist. Consequently the Ancient Aryans set immense store on fitness and strength.'[16]

Alongside the bilge about the ancient Aryan origins of yoga, *About Yoga* touches on the usual obsessions of the genre. It is broken down into chapters on subjects such as hygiene, diet, sleep, emotions and breathing. When it comes to the latter topic, Day was clearly influenced by the previously mentioned fake guru Ramacharaka, aka William Walker Atkinson, whose books are listed in *About Yoga*'s bibliography.[17] Ultimately, Day's book is as much about health, happiness and living a long life as it is about yoga specifically. This (lack of) focus reflects how many of the other yoga books listed in the bibliography and discussed later in this chapter were constructed and marketed. Day, however, goes a step further than most on the matter of long life by offering the lure of immortality:

> I believe with the yogis, that there is no such thing as 'natural death.' Death is unnatural and it is inevitable only because Man has lost the secret of eternal life. I have spoken with yogis who seemed to be able to control some of the laws of nature, and they have told me that anyone who masters yoga thoroughly can live on indefinitely.[18]

While Day isn't the only writer of yoga books to explicitly claim it is possible to live to be hundreds of years old, most authors with an uncritical faith in the occult capacity of *asanas* and breathing exercises at least hold back from stating this in print. That said, it was clearly something a considerable cross-section of the twentieth-century yoga book readership wanted to hear.

About Yoga enjoyed sufficient success for Day's publisher to issue a follow-up work within two years. *The Study And*

Practice Of Yoga, published in 1953 acts as a manual for those wanting to do *asanas* and draws on authors such as Sivananda Saraswati, whose *Yogic Home Exercises* is included in the previous book's bibliography.[19] After sitting poses and breathing exercises, Day recommends starting *asanas* with *surya namaskars*, aka sun salutations.[20] This makes him appear more advanced in his yoga practice than many of the other authors mentioned thus far, as sun salutations were at the time not widely known in Anglo-American yoga. Even so, it may simply be that he cobbled together his yoga programme from what he had read elsewhere rather than having a set practice himself, as Day was first and foremost a jobbing hack. This is backed up by his somewhat cynical remark in *You, Too, Can Write For Money*: 'Given that little bit of extra knowledge on any subject, you can start writing a book on it. By the time your research and preparation for the book are finished, *you will probably be an expert*, too.'[21]

As already mentioned, the bibliography in *About Yoga*, while short, provides a useful snapshot of the various yoga and occult books that had caught Day's eye in the preceding years and thus presumably had some degree of influence at the time. In terms of the supposed Eastern origins of the yogic traditions, aside from two works each by Francis Yeats-Brown, Alexander Cannon and William Walker Atkinson (under his Ramacharaka pen name), there are three works by Paul Brunton, two by Alexandra David-Neel, and one each by H. P. Blavatsky and Theos Bernard, as well as an anthology of Tibetan yoga texts in translation with commentaries by W. Y. Evans-Wentz. These, alongside translations of Hindu religious texts and commentaries on them, suggest that Day's knowledge of the 'Mystic East' was heavily reliant on Western discourse provided by lightweight academic texts, yellow-press journalism and the writing of outright charlatans.[22] In short, he was drawn to popular authors on occultism and Eastern mysticism, whose works are not generally viewed as reliable or scientific.

In terms of books about yoga more generally, *About Yoga*'s bibliography kicks off with Claude Bragdon's *Yoga For You*, published prior to the end of the Second World War.[23] Bragdon (1866–1946) was an American architect with an amateur interest in spiritualism and oriental philosophy. As he writes in the Preface to his earlier *An Introduction To Yoga*:[24]

> I have never taken lessons in Yoga, much less given them. I have never been to India; nor can I lay claim to that order of scholarship based on exhaustive knowledge which makes possible the deciphering and comparison of texts. I have read only those books — and them uncritically — which would fall naturally into the hands of anyone interested in Oriental philosophy ... but there is another side to the picture ... I have met many Hindus in the course of my life and number several among my friends. All of them knew something about Yoga either at first or at second hand ... To them Yoga was a *living* thing ... Something of this livingness I have tried to recapture and render here.[25]

In other words, Bragdon's approach to critical scholarship appears largely to consist of accepting what he reads and taking the word of those he talks to. Nevertheless, Bragdon's *Yoga For You* is considerably more bizarre than his first work, with the author claiming to have composed it after being contacted by a 'Delphic Woman' who told him: 'I was to write another book, a last testament in which I should bequeath to the generation now growing up whatever helpful wisdom I had to give.'[26] Moreover, the book includes passages supposedly written by a being from another plane called the 'Brown Brother'. While Bragdon is more interested in mental cleansing than modern postural practice, he does mention a few *asanas* in his chapters on 'Posture' and 'Exercise'.[27] Inevitably, there are chapters on chakras and breathing, alongside warnings about the dangers of the *incubi* and *succubi*, sexual demons who drain people of their energies during sleep. Overall, Bragdon's book comes across as surrealist fiction depicting a man in the throes of a psychotic delusion. As such, it is telling that Day refers to Bragdon in his bibliography, but it does give a sense of the reliability – or lack thereof – of the source material being used by popular authors of yoga texts at the time. Bragdon takes this to an extreme, highlighting the ways most writing on yoga, both then and now, is saturated with occultism.

The madcap nature of Bragdon's work at least makes him more entertaining than most of the authors who claim to have travelled to India and conversed with gurus there. One such individual mentioned in Day's bibliography – for their short 1940 book *Tantrik Yoga: Hindu & Tibetan* – is infamous antisemite and Nazi collaborator, J. Marquès-Rivière (pen name of Jean-Marie Rivière, 1903–2000).[28] Condemned to death in absentia for his wartime activities,[29] Marquès-Rivière found refuge in Francoist Spain. In the mentioned book, much space is devoted to Hindu notions of the subtle body and the *chakras*, with – despite the title – a mere page or so given over to Tibetan traditions.

Another book listed in Day's bibliography is *The Inner Tradition And Yoga* by Charles Wase, which stands as another prime example of Eastern mysticism being used to add spice to Western esoteric traditions. Here alchemy, breathing exercises and occidental mysticism are topped with some Hindu sweeteners, with cultural specificity set aside in favour of a belief that East and West offer alternative paths to a single 'perennial philosophy'. To be more specific: 'The two methods of training do not really clash, because the Eastern method is, in one sense, more deeply spiritual, contemplative and individual and passive: whereas the Western method is more in the nature of a system of training in right-thinking and the more active process of positive thought ... Both schools are correct.'[30]

Other books in Day's bibliography with somewhat self-explanatory titles include *Extra-Sensory Perception* by J. B. Rhine and *Gland Treatment For Renewal Or Rejuvenation Of The Body Through Applied New Thought* by Grace Stuart.[31] Meanwhile, Felix Guyot (1880–1960) features twice in Day's bibliography. The more revealing of his two tomes is *Yoga For The West*, published in the first half of the 1930s, which is pitched at those wishing to become occult initiates.[32] Guyot's description of non-physical initiatory training systems begins with various optional Western esoteric exercises that do not form part of the Eastern system he is most concerned with. Having done so, he moves on to his recommended psychic training, claiming that students should follow a religion – if necessary, choosing one off the peg if they don't already adhere to a creed – in order to sustain them. He counsels:

> ... it is not a matter of believing, but of acting as though you did believe ... As regards the religion to be chosen, we think that the best are the Jewish religion as set forth in the Cabala, and the Roman Catholic religion, in its esoteric aspect, about which very many books have been written. For those whose tastes incline them towards the East, Buddhism and especially Hinduism are to be recommended. Finally, Free Masonry can very adequately take the place of religion.[33]

In other words, the reader needn't be particularly fussy in their spiritual beliefs. Moving on, some of Guyot's exercises entail refusing to see what is in front of one's eyes, while purporting to witness the impossible – perhaps an appropriate analogy for much of modern yoga: 'when the image of an envelope disappears both from the consciousness and the infra-astral vision, one can read what is inside the envelope.'[34]

Even if the specific exercises may be unfamiliar to the contemporary reader, their general tenor and the results sought from them will be familiar to anyone with a passing interest in other twentieth-century systems of occult development. For example, one exercise consists of holding your arm out bent, then through imagining it is straight convincing yourself this is the reality.[35] This is exactly the type of training later writers such as Frank Rudolph Young – who developed a system of exercise he called 'Yogametrics' – suggest for occult development (see Chapter 13). Likewise, the stress Guyot's system places on relaxation, breathing, some physical exercises and numerous mental concentration exercises (aka meditation) is replicated in the later Yogism system of Paul Brunton's (an early populariser of neo-Hindu spiritualism) associates at the Insight School of Yoga.

While, as previously detailed, there is a strong case for asserting modern postural practice originated in the US, it was Indian nationalists who produced the most impressive early yoga manuals. This is reflected in Day's bibliography, which lists a slightly late arrival among these guidebooks: astrologer V. G. Rele's 1939 volume *Yogic Asanas*, which was a follow-up to *The Mysterious Kundalini* (also listed in the bibliography).[36] In *Yogic Asanas*, Rele asserts:

> Yogic physical culture, unlike many Western systems of physical culture, does not make a pretence of merely developing the superficial muscles of the body, but the exercises do make them healthy and strong, particularly the trunk muscles, by requisitioning their help to tone up all the involuntary organs of the body which are mainly concerned with such processes as digestion, evacuation, circulation, res-

piration and secretion, and through them the autonomic nervous system which regulates their activities.[37]

These claims mirror the earlier rhetoric of F. A. Hornibrook (1877–1965), whose 1924 work *The Culture of the Abdomen* features in the bibliographies of both *Yogic Asanas* and Harvey Day's *The Study And Practice Of Yoga*.[38] In his book, Hornibrook positively contrasts his easy exercise system – which definitively *isn't* modern postural practice – to competing health programmes:

> It is common knowledge that by constant use muscle becomes larger and harder, and on that foundation of imperfect knowledge have been built up the various erroneous systems of bodily culture seen in gymnasia all over the world. These systems have, as their aim, group or regional development, the attention being chiefly focused unto the limb groups, while the trunk is ignored[39]

The focus of *The Culture of the Abdomen* is on curing constipation, eating less and not wearing restrictive clothing, all themes taken up by many of the later 'yogis' mentioned in this chapter. This points to the fact that rather than providing something markedly different to nineteenth- and twentieth-century Western physical and health culture, modern postural practice in fact drew on and then displaced established occidental systems, in part through a rebranding exercise that sold what was on offer as an 'exotic' Indian import. Mark Singleton, despite drawing on a different set of sources and practices than those used here, makes an analogous argument in his book, *Yoga Body*.[40]

Shifting back from the books Harvey Day plundered for material to Day himself, the hack journalist continued to churn out books on yoga, food and diet, cricket and the occult until just a few years before his death at the age of 89.[41] The many publications Day penned features for included *Prediction*, a magazine discussed in the next chapter.[42] Back in the 1950s, Day's first two yoga books seem to have made him his publisher's key modern postural practice author of the time — his works are advertised on the dust jackets of several other books published by Thorsons, including Alain's *Yoga For Perfect Health* and Major P. G. Francis's *Yoga The Amazing Life Science*.[43] Not only does the wide circulation of Day's books and writing make him a far more important figure in the development of British yoga in the second half of the twentieth century than he is generally credited with, the various writers he cites in his work provide evidence of which pre-Second World War influences had come to saturate contemporary ideas on postural practice.

11

Desmond Dunne aka Occultist James Lee-Richardson and His Mail Order Yoga Course

Publishing yoga books at the same time as Day, and also claiming to be adapting the practice to contemporary Western needs, was Desmond Dunne, aka James Lee-Richardson (1913–85). As a young man, Lee-Richardson began his publishing career as a journalist and editor using the pseudonym James Leigh. It was under this name that he compiled the 1936 *Manual And Who's Who Of Spiritualism And Psychic Research*, the title page of which refers to him as the editor of occultist magazine *Prediction*.[1] Lee-Richardson not only sold mail order yoga instruction, but flogged courses on tarot, palm reading, astrology and psychic development from his home in the south-west London suburbs.[2] To fully understand what Lee-Richardson brought to yoga and where he was running with it, it is necessary to delve into his panoply of crank obsessions, many of which cross over into the occult, as well as his many business hustles, which foreshadow the multi-billion industry modern postural yoga has become.

Likewise, Lee-Richardson's business activities can be seen as a precursor to those of Alex Jones of Infowars infamy, albeit without the hate content. As we will see below, like Jones, Lee-Richardson built a media empire peddling fake news. Both men used their publishing operations to shift income-generating health supplements.[3] The range of issues covered by Lee-Richardson's media outlets was broader than that of Jones, and the former covered many subjects – such as UFOs – whose boosters, like Jones, were prone to stray into conspiracy theory.

As a result of his yoga-related activities, Lee-Richardson – or rather his Desmond Dunne persona – was grandiosely promoted on the dust jacket of his 1951 book *Yoga For Everyman* as 'the world's most successful teacher of yoga'.[4] Lee-Richardson makes for an interesting contrast to Day, as he keeps his occult interests closer to his chest in his books – seemingly saving such information for those prepared to shell out for his mail order courses.[5]

In his books, Lee-Richardson's claims about the life-extending possibilities of yoga are relatively modest compared to Day's assertions: he suggests yoga can be used to live to 100 years old.[6] Nevertheless, if the claims of his publisher are to be believed, he had just as much, perhaps more, influence on how yoga – and by extension modern postural practice – came to be perceived in the West during the post-war era. As such, it is worth taking the time to scratch below the surface of what Lee-Richardson presents in his books.

In *Yoga For Everyman*, Lee-Richardson describes his modern adaptation of yoga as 'yogism', which he outlines as consisting of very basic relaxation, contraction, breathing and concentration (aka basic meditation) exercises. Many, if not all, of these exercises appear to have been inspired at least in part by Felix Guyot. Despite the book being a relatively slim 116 pages, this still leaves considerable space for filler, including instructions on how best to make compost heaps.[7] Towards the end of the book are a series of drawings and descriptions of *asanas* that bear the somewhat ominous disclaimer: 'regular practice of Deep Contraction obviates the necessity of assuming more difficult postures. Many of the historic poses are quite unsuited to Western use. This list below is given solely for historic interest.'⁸ What follows is a fairly standard selection of *asanas* – aside from peacock, most are regularly taught in gym yoga classes today.

Turning to Lee-Richardson's mail order Insight School of Yoga course, the first lesson is contained within a blue wrapper on which are printed positive assessments of yoga from, amongst others, our old enemy Major F. Yeats-Brown, Thomas Mann (novelist), Sir Francis Younghusband (Knight Commander of the Indian Empire), Madam Call-Curci (singer) and Julian Huxley (evolutionary biologist). Here, the quote provided by Shaw Desmond (1877–1960) – described as 'the famous author', although he is now largely forgotten – takes us to a new level of absurdity when it comes to pseudo-historical claims about yoga: 'Kant, Hegel, Max Müller, all world-famous names, were interested or actual followers of Yoga. Pythagoras, Plato, Descartes and Spinoza were all believers in Yoga and therefore, in Yoga breathing and prana.'⁹ Within the lessons, Lee-Richardson makes similar far-fetched historical assertions to those he attributes to Shaw Desmond, although he provides no sources for them: 'The Greek thinkers were the first Europeans to discover and develop Metaphysics … Later research has proved that much of this Wisdom was brought from India by those who went with Alexander's conquering Army, and some of it trickled through even before the advent of Alexander.'¹⁰ Here, it is worth noting that both Pythagoras and Plato – the supposed 'believers in yoga' – died before Alexander the Great's ultimately unsuccessful invasion of the Indian subcontinent.

While there is overlap between the Insight course and *Yoga For Everyman*, it is apparent that the former contains a good deal of material intended for a more 'select' audience. Among other things, the course attempts to convince its participants that they will be made privy to secret occult teachings: 'Of course it would be useless to seek this secret knowledge without tuition. Yogism is the best of all Teachers since it brings you the combined work of leading eastern AND western Yogis, scientists, psychologists and medical men, who have worked side by side to perfect it.'[11] This passage, taken from the first lesson, seems to imply the course was put together collectively by a group of relevant experts. It isn't until the concluding *Lesson XII* that Dunne finally signs off at the end with his (fake) name, thereby revealing he is solely responsible for the mysteries that have been unveiled. Underneath his signature is a stern reminder that 'You have given an undertaking not to divulge these Lessons to any other person.'[12] The first lesson makes some grand promises as to what it will deliver to the eager student:

> ... your study of Yogism will help you earn more money, gain the promotion of your private plans, and liberate your life from crippling anxieties ... Yogism will develop the psychic or intuitive side of your nature, so that you will know the inspiration available to all who unfold their inner faculties. Here again western science lags behind a thousand years. In our modern universities the vital faculties of clairvoyance and telepathy are just now being rediscovered[13]

The Insight School of Yoga offered the gradual revelation of occult 'wisdom' to those willing to commit themselves fully to the course (as well as shell out for it). In this, Lee-Richardson's mail order instruction has parallels to Freemasonry as filtered through organisations such as the Hermetic Order of the Golden Dawn. There are also sly indications that Lee-Richardson himself is a Mason, such as references to God in Masonic terms: 'The Great Architect designed your spine so that there is a curve forward in the neck.'[14] More generally, the idea of secret knowledge to be learned in due course is a recurring trope in the course. In *Lesson II*, for example, under the heading 'Secrets of Yoga Breathing', the text instructs the reader:

> ... don't be impatient to learn about individual aspects of Yoga which may have some immediate attraction for you. And don't waste your time reading books or literature on the subject. This you can do to much better advantage later, when the initial ground has been covered.[15]

Here, a cynic might argue that if students were to read other material at the same time, they might hit upon the texts – especially those of Aleister Crowley and Felix Guyot – that the Insight School so clearly draws on. By delaying any wider reading, Lee-Richardson also buys time to mould his student's views, meaning contrary opinions that may be encountered later are more likely to be rejected out of hand. At the very end of the course, the Insight School generously provides a set of approved resources for further study (with Lee-Richardson's various mail order occult courses being strongly recommended). Before students get there, however, they are subjected to a variety of dogmatic, occultist assertions about yoga that leave any critical thinking on the subject at the door. For example, *Lesson II* claims that:

> There is an elixir in the air which no machine, however delicate, has been able to weigh or measure – and no machine ever will. The Yogis call it Prana and it is this which has such a great sedative effect and which makes us conscious of occult forces if we persevere in breathing it in the Yogic way.[16]

This sets up those following the course for the more dangerous pseudo-scientific claims on personal health that crop up in the next lesson: 'If you breathe in the right way, you can avoid illness. You need never have catarrh, and you can banish all dread of tuberculosis, which cannot touch you if you breathe correctly. It is even possible that such diseases as gangrene are due to defective breathing.'[17]

Baseless assertions of this type had been floating around yogic discourses for decades, and more recently have fed into the embrace of anti-vax ideologies by many of those involved with modern postural practice, particularly in the wake of the Covid-19 pandemic.[18] The same lesson also offers much else that is scientifically questionable:

> One can never develop psychic qualities in a gross or sensual body. Nor in an unclean body, and that is why so much stress is being laid on cleanliness ... At a later stage some of the secrets of rejuvenation will be divulged – and even after a Course of twelve lessons it will be possible for you to prolong your life considerably.[19]

Such claims, which draw on the bodily purity tropes seen in much of the fascist yoga previously discussed (and which mirror discourses about racial purity), seem custom-made to appeal to the desperate and credulous. *Lesson IV* continues the 'psychic' infantilisation of those taking the course with pie-in-the-sky lines such as 'the mystic word "OM" has mysterious power and will greatly strengthen the forces you are awakening within yourself' and 'you can concentrate on relatives and friends ... This power of concentration will ultimately develop into telepathy.'[20]

Later, *Lesson VI* provides '15 New Commandments of Health of Mind and Body', supposedly based on early Yoga texts.[21] In reality, these 'new commandments' appear to be more influenced by New Thought and Freemasonry – both of which are rooted in Christianity – than classical Hindu yoga. The following lessons continue in a similar vein, with a few basic *asanas* incorporated into sets of daily exercises, accompanied by a steady stream of pseudo-science and pseudo-history, not to mention regular invocation of the Bible and biblical figures.

Overall, it seems to me likely that Lee-Richardson – like Felix Guyot before him – set out to draw others into a deeply religious programme of 'self-development', with the promise of psychic powers deployed primarily as a way of selling this. My conclusion that *Yoga For Everyman* provides an 'outer' teaching designed to draw some but not all its readers to an 'inner' teaching is diametrically opposed to Suzanne Newcombe's contention in *Yoga In Britain*, that Lee-Richardson helped make a secular form of yoga more acceptable in the initial post-war period.[22]

Aside from Lee-Richardson's occult involvements, he was very much a businessman and salesman. While, judging by the amount of time he devoted to spiritualism and other occult pursuits, Lee-Richardson was a true believer, this didn't stop him deploying hype and manipulation to extract money from those who shared his interests. In this, like everyone else, he was living out the contradictions of capitalism.

In her book, Newcombe refers to Lee-Richardson's use of the British social research organisation Mass Observation, again seemingly without questioning his motivation:

> Dunne paid the British social research organization Mass-Observation (MO) to interview 'a representative cross-section of the public in a London district about their reactions to life' and reported the responses in his book *Yoga for Everyman* (1951). The MO questions focused on discovering how much of the general population was affected by 'a lack of energy, frustration, the sense of purposelessness' – problems which Dunne believed could be alleviated through his system of Yogism.[23]

Given Lee-Richardson as a businessman had a use for both market research and advertising material – the comments from Mass Observation could provide something analogous to a celebrity endorsement – it seems probable that he commissioned the MO surveys for these purposes. That said, the possibility that he simply claimed to have commissioned the surveys without actually doing so cannot entirely be discounted.[24] Lee-Richardson also claimed he asked 'Mass-Observation to undertake a second inquiry. This was directed to results reported by people who were actually studying Yogism ... One thousand reports voluntarily submitted by students of the School of Yoga were accordingly analysed.'[25] In a 1955 UK advert for the School of Yoga, a selection of endorsements from students concludes: 'Thousands of similar tributes verified by Mass Observation. Let Yogism help you.'[26] Here, note the inflation from the previously reported 'thousand' students to the 'multiple thousands' four years later. The Insight School of Yoga also published advertisements for sample lessons. Once a punter was lured in with these, they were presumably given the hard sell on the more expensive complete mail order course. While print runs are hard to estimate, given that the Insight School had international offices and produced an advanced course, it appears the mail order course sold well.

Lee-Richardson's second book using the Dunne pseudonym, *The Manual Of Yoga*, doesn't contain much that isn't in his previous tome.[27] In the book, published in 1956, Lee-Richardson states: 'I do not advise you, as I have said before, to adopt the Head-stand asana (Sirsasana); unless you happen to be a professional acrobat.'[28] This assertion, however, is completely contradicted in his later 1961 book *Yoga Made Easy*:

Sirshasana, or *The Headstand*, traditionally associated with Yoga and second only to Lotus or Buddha Pose in identifying the entire subject of Hatha Yoga in the Western mind. It is not nearly as difficult to do as people imagine, may be learned at any age and, once mastered, is wonderfully relaxing and all-inclusive.[29]

This turnaround on performing headstands appears to stem at least in part from a salesman's desire to tell people what they want to hear, and was probably dictated by the fact that there was an increasing amount of easily accessible information about yoga in print, depicting headstand as a key part of the discipline. As such, Lee-Richardson was obliged to move with the times. While much of the content of *Yoga Made Easy* is recycled from Lee-Richardson's earlier books and mail order yoga courses, the way it is presented by the publisher indicates a desire to appeal to a mass-market American audience. This can be seen in the bold declaration on the front cover: 'In this book, the ancient Asian discipline of yoga is adapted to the American way of life – to let you benefit from nature's own way of maintaining physical and mental health.' The author biography on the inside back flap further backs this up, claiming that *Yoga Made Easy* in particular 'is especially suited to the American way of life', and that Dunne 'is also the publisher of numerous magazines dealing with Physical well-being, including *Fate* and *Here's Health* … Desmond Dunne is Principal of the world-wide School of Yoga. He has taught the subject to thousands of people in the branches of his school in New Zealand, Norway, Switzerland, Belgium, Morocco and France.'

In further unravelling Lee-Richardson's business and occult connections, it is illuminating to take a closer look at the credits on the magazines being published from the Manor House, Worcester Park, Surrey, address that pops up in his sign-off as 'Desmond Dunne' to *The Manual Of Yoga*. Lee-Richardson is credited under his James Leigh pseudonym as editor of the British edition of occult magazine *Fate*, one of the associate editors of which is Adrienne Arden.[30] Arden was also the principal of the Insight Institute, Insight House, 132 Malden Road, New Malden, Surrey, England (Lee-Richardson's business address in the late 1940s and early 1950s) – known after moving its base of operations to nearby Worcester Park as the Insight Institute School of Personal Analysis and Development.[31] In other words, this is a parallel business to Lee-Richardson's Insight School of Yoga and was run from the same addresses as his other commercial activities. It seems likely that Arden was made principal of the Insight Institute because her *News of the World* astrology column made her the most widely recognised name associated with this business venture.

Alongside Arden, the Directors of Studies at the Insight Institute were 'Richard Eden, Noel Jaquin, Colin Evans, Edward Whitman, Vera Crompton and Frank Lind', all of whom worked for *Prediction* magazine and other occult publications.[32] Lind was later replaced by another *Prediction* columnist and high-profile occultist Madeline Montalban.[33] *Prediction*'s first editor was Lee-Richardson under his James Leigh pseudonym,[34] although he appears to have given up editorship of the magazine to focus on his own publishing business in 1953. The biographies of the various directors of the institute are revealing.

Noel Jacquin authored a series of books about palm reading and had established himself as a leading writer on the subject in the 1920s; Frank Lind wrote a regular column for *Prediction* entitled 'Occult Case Book', an anthology of which was collected as *My Occult Case Book* in 1953, with an introduction by James Leigh.[35] Vera Compton was the author of *Palmistry For Everyone* (1952),[36] and Edward Whitman later penned a three-volume work on astrology subtitled *Astro-Kinetics*. It is unclear who Colin Evans was given how common the name is, but it may have been the fraudulent medium of that name whose claimed ability to levitate has been widely debunked.[37] Richard Eden's identity requires further investigation, as it seems possible this could be one of Lee-Richardson's pseudonyms, with the moniker possibly taken from the Tudor alchemist, translator and English imperialist Richard Eden (c.1520–76). Madeline Montalban, meanwhile, was associated with all the best-known UK occultists and witches of her era from Aleister Crowley on down, and ran her own mail order occult initiation course. Given the interests of the various directors, it should come as little surprise that the Insight Institute offered mail order courses on, among other things, astrology, palmistry, graphology and psychic powers.[38]

The association between yoga and this motley crew of occultists dates back to the very inception of *Prediction* in 1936, with the word 'yoga' featuring on the covers of the magazine's March, April, May, June, July, September and October issues.[39] The July issue also features a three-page article by Paul Brunton entitled 'I Interview An Indian Yogi! My Meeting With The Most Famous Occultist In All India':

> When I first came here more than five years ago, I had the privilege of having many private chats with the Sage (Maharishee), wherein many problems were solved, but since my return to him last November, our communication has been almost entirely silent and telepathic … I have seen him perfectly clearly, in what people would call astral or clairvoyant vision, on several occasions during my travels in the West.[40]

The same issue also carried a feature entitled 'Strange Feats Of The Yogis' by Pundit Dinkarswami, which describes a yogi bringing a dead man back to life, as well as an article by famed American author and political activist Upton Sinclair entitled 'How I Discovered Telepathy'.[41] In fact, the magazine, despite its esoteric focus, managed to attract many famous names of the time.

Overall, there can be little doubt about Lee-Richardson's deep immersion in the occult, nor that his Insight School of Yoga course was just one example of his many hustles. Another element of Lee-Richardson's operations were his UK *Here's Health* publications. Scattered throughout the 1959 *Here's Health Family Guide* and on the back page are ads for his supplement business Healthcrafts, purveyors of vitamin and herbal pills that purportedly help with ailments ranging from menopause to constipation, and from feeling tired and run down to obesity.[42] Lee-Richardson may not have been the first person to discover peddling fake news was a good marketing hook on which to sell quack health products, but he was doing so decades before Alex Jones' Infowars operation.

All of the above also suggests that Lee-Richardson's story offers an instructive example on how influential figures are either written out of the history of modern postural practice, or never written into it in the first place, as they don't fit the preconceptions of editors and journalists addressing the subject of yoga. Lee-Richardson appears to have no direct connection to India, which many of those who comment on modern postural practice assume is its home. Through the use of pen names, he also shunned personal publicity. It is a common mistake of our celebrity-obsessed culture to treat fame and influence as synonymous, when they are often quite distinct. Lee-Richardson devoted much more of his time to making money as a businessman flogging yoga courses around the world than teaching postural practice, which to those who look at capitalist society empirically might indicate more – rather than less – influence on its spread.

During the twentieth century, mail order courses played a key role in the global reception of many exercise and occult systems, with the iconic Charles Atlas body-building system an obvious go-to illustration of this. Lee-Richardson's businesses provide another pre-eminent example. As such, he should be treated as far more than a mere footnote to the history of modern yoga and occultism.

12
Richard Hittleman and Yogic Televangelism

Richard Hittleman (1927–91) had a range of yoga-focused business interests that may not have been as varied as those of James Lee-Richardson, but this yoga televangelist was still an accomplished cod-spiritual salesman. Hittleman didn't need to diversify in the way Lee-Richardson did because he was Mr Yoga in the Anglo-American world of modern postural practice. Over the course of his career, Hittleman demonstrated that it was possible to be as backward as those yogis peddling occult pseudo-science, whether of a fascist or non-fascist persuasion, by pushing a very different faith-based approach to modern postural practice.

Hittleman became a minor television personality in the 1960s and 1970s by hosting both US and UK yoga instruction shows, and also put together publications and records along similar lines, some of which he sold directly to the public. Hittleman may not quite have had the Mr Showbiz reputation of Ed Sullivan, but he had far greater audience reach than anyone else with a yoga TV programme. He was, according to his ex-wife Linda Hittleman, 'very private'.[1] This desire for privacy is reflected in the lack of autobiographical information contained within his books. In this respect, the introduction to his 1968 book *Guide To Yoga Meditation* is about as good as it gets. Hittlemen begins by briefly outlining his early experiences with yoga:

> When experimenting with certain methods of general instruction at Columbia University Teachers College, I discovered quite by accident that a bare minimum of Yoga practices performed by my fellow students and teachers ... produced some very dramatic results ... Classes which I taught personally during the 1940s and 50s were well attended and I had the opportunity to work closely with many hundreds of students.

Having done so, he describes in broad strokes his rise to small-screen fame:

> In 1961 I conceived of Yoga instruction through a television series to reach the population *en masse* ... While the series was still in the planning stages, one of the production company's executives said to me, 'Your presentation is fine and we think the exercises are excellent. But couldn't you call them anything other than Yoga?' This was in 1961. The 'foreign' stigma was still in full effect. This year [1968] while discussing the format for a television 'special' which would deal solely with aspects of Yoga in the United States, a network official said to me, 'But couldn't you allow your hair to grow long and wear some robes? You just don't look like a Hindu!' Thus, within one decade, Yoga in America would appear to have come full circle.[2]

While providing a great example of Hittleman pitching himself as a misunderstood 'genius' whose timing had been proved right, little concrete biographical detail is provided. Hittleman was also cagey about how, when and where he learned yoga, as the following exchange from his book *Guide For The Seeker* illustrates:

> *Student*: Do you have – or did you have – a guru?

RH: All who pushed me from outside and forced me to turn inwards have been my gurus.

Student: I mean, was there a particular guru?

RH: I know what you mean ... Ramana Maharshi.

Student: Can you tell us some of your experiences?

RH: No. It is not my way to speak of these things. There are those who do recount experiences with their gurus.[3]

Elsewhere, there are scattered references to Hittleman learning yoga during childhood. Howard Kent, in his introduction to *Yoga For Health*, says: 'Richard Hittleman first learned of Yoga when he was an eight-year-old child living on the East Coast of America',[4] while Ami Chen Mills in her 'Death and Taxes' posthumous profile of Hittleman asserts that 'Hittleman learned yoga from his parent's Hindu maintenance man at a getaway called Utopia in the Catskills'.[5] In terms of *asana* practice, Suzanne Newcombe speculates: 'Hittleman was not too far away from Pierre Bernard's Nyack Country Club and it is also possible that he had contact with yoga through members of this group, or other teachers in New York City.'[6] Meanwhile, the author blurbs on the back covers of Hittleman's first two books claim that he 'spent several years in secluded study with Hindu Yogis after he graduated from Columbia University Teachers College'.[7]

Here, it is worth noting that Ramana Maharshi, who Hittleman names as his guru above, had very little interest in postural yoga, so it seems debatable whether Hittleman learnt much from him on the subject – if indeed his years of 'secluded study' actually took place. Given that Hittleman likely completed his teacher training in his early twenties, and that Maharishi was sick with cancer from 1948 onwards and died in April 1950, this would not have afforded the world's leading yoga televangelist much opportunity to study with his stated guru. On the other hand, Paul Brunton – another of Maharshi's Western disciples – claimed to be able to communicate telepathically with his guru, so perhaps Hittleman's physical presence wasn't required. In this respect, when asked in *Guide For The Seeker* is 'your physical presence necessary for this type of initiation?', Hittleman responds: 'No. Those who practice Yoga seriously by using my books and recordings, or through the instruction I offer on my television programs, know of my presence.'[8] In other words, purchasing his yogic 'product' or engaging with it on TV offers sufficient substitute for being in his physical presence.

Beyond hype about the efficacy of yoga as a health system, Hittleman's Prentice Hall instruction manuals are generally somewhat dry, bereft of the more outrageous occult baloney peddled by the likes of Indra Devi and Frank Rudolph Young. Hittleman's rationale for this is made explicit in his later *Guide To Meditation*:

> ... the *physical* properties of Yoga were stressed in this era of instruction, the supposition on the part of the teachers being: If the student were drawn into the physical practice the health benefits would be so pronounced that he would then desire to learn *more of the philosophy* and to practice the *meditation* techniques; these were, after all, the entire 'essence' of the subject.[9]

As this implies, Hittleman's outer physical culture teachings promoting youthfulness and health were used as a means of drawing students to his inner teachings, which were in fact faith-based and anti-science from beginning to end. The lack of a scientific basis for the supposed health benefits of yoga as propounded by Hittleman can be seen in, for example, his first book *Be Young With Yoga*, published in 1962, which carries the strap-line, 'The Amazing 7-Week Course in Yoga that

Stimulates Your Body with Fresh Vitality and the Bubbling Energy of Youth':

> The publicity given the HEAD STAND in connection with Yoga ... is justified, not as a peculiarity but as a tremendously dynamic technique that has the most marvellous effect on the brain. Make every attempt to perfect the HEAD STAND; it may take time but it is well worth your efforts.[10]

No scientific evidence is offered to back up this claim. While headstands may be a staple of the yoga world and fun to perform, there are many other exercises that more efficiently promote health, well-being and functional balance (freestanding on a Swiss ball to name but one). Hittleman's second book, *Yoga For Physical Fitness*, which appeared two years later, carries the strap-line: 'Easy-to-do coordination, strengthening and isometric Yoga exercises especially designed for office workers and housewives.' Although isometric exercises – in which muscles are simply flexed, with no joint movement made – had long been used in both strength training and martial arts, during the 1960s they became something of a fad following the publication of research by Theodor Hettinger and Erich Albert Müller at the Max Planck Institute in Germany. As such, it is unsurprising to see them invoked as a selling point. Despite the gentle, 'easy-to-do' sales pitch, quite a number of the exercises in the book (and in many other yoga manuals) are not considered safe from a sports science perspective. For example, *Yoga For Physical Fitness* includes full neck rolls, which put undue pressure on the cervical spine.[11]

While Hittleman's Prentice Hall books enjoyed widespread trade distribution, 'seekers' could also order booklets and records direct from the yoga televangelist himself. The 40-page pamphlet *Yoga Philosophy & Meditation: An Interpre-*

tation is typical in this regard, offering proof that Hittleman's modern postural practice was simply a gateway into a world of radically anti-scientific superstitions:

> Whereas we have been led to accept the theory that man has somehow evolved from a more primitive creature and that civilisation may be approximately 7,000 years old, the Yogi would comment on the former statement as 'absurd' and the latter statement as 'yesterday'![12]

In other words, in a similar vein to many Christian fundamentalists, Hittleman rejects the theory of evolution in favour of religious cosmology. Sadly this was not a passing phase, but rather part and parcel of his deep-rooted anti-science ideology. The passage just quoted is repeated word-for-word five years later in Hittleman's 1969 book *Guide To Yoga Meditation*, which also adds such useful resources as a picture of 'The 7 centers of force which are opened through the journey of the Basic Power' – a reference to a mythological 'kundalini power' that lights the equally non-existent 'chakras' in the human body.[13] In a foreshadowing of the anti-vaccine movement that came to particular prominence during the Covid-19 pandemic, Hittleman makes repeated references to a 'conspiracy' when peddling his anti-science line on evolution in later works. For instance, in *Yoga: The 8 Steps To Health And Peace*, he asserts:

> The ordinary mind, in its endless and futile speculations as to its own origins, has relatively recently developed a theory of man's 'evolution.' This new ingredient of the mayic conspiracy, currently accepted by a large segment of the world's population, postulates that man has *reached* (evolved into) his present state of advanced (but imperfect) development through a series of transformations: microbe,

fish and ape are some of the stops along the way. In the context of Yoga this theory cannot claim our attention for more than a moment.[14]

In fact, the first part of the book is titled 'The Great Conspiracy', with Chapter 3 ('Dis-Illusionment: Exposing The Conspiracy'), making the case that 'The true guru is the great dis-illusioner. Throughout the ages he has blown the whistle on the conspiracy; he has explained the nature of maya.'[15] To spell it out, to Hittleman, science is '*maya*' or 'illusion', preventing seekers from discovering the 'truth'. Here, it is also worth pointing out that in Hittleman's conservative, patriarchal worldview, a guru is inevitably male.

Despite adopting a primarily faith-based approach to yoga, there are several curious affinities between Hittleman and yoga occultists such as Claude Bragdon (dealt with in Chapter 10 above), with the former appearing to tell a variation of a story previously recounted by the latter on how to become a successful 'seeker'. Bragdon's version is more specific, stating that 'My friend Dan Gopal Mukerji told me once, when a boy, while bathing with his mother's *guru* in the Ganges, that good, wise, and usually kindly old man suddenly seized him by the hair and held his head under water until he was nearly suffocated.'[16] Hittleman, by contrast, is vaguer, stating only that 'There is the story of the master [guru] and his student who were sitting at the edge of a river and discussing the practice necessary to achieve enlightenment.' The story proceeds thus:

> The master grasped his student about the neck and held his head beneath the water. The student struggled to release himself but the master held him firmly. Finally the master pulled his head from the water and released him. The student gulped air into his lungs. Then the master said to him: 'When I held you under, what was the uppermost

thing in your mind?' 'Air, air' gasped the student. 'Exactly so must you crave enlightenment' stated the master.[17]

The seeming indifference to abusive behaviour spotlighted in this story is integral to the self-image of religious detachment Hittleman attempted to project. As his ex-wife Linda later observed, Hittleman wished at all times to be seen as 'a spiritual guy. That was how he became a religion.'[18] In reality, the wisdom he dispensed is on a par with that you might expect from a mediocre motivational coach, and is just as applicable to making money as it is to achieving 'enlightenment'. This is apparent from the fact that the story told above has since been reworked by management gurus as the made-up tale of Socrates half-drowning a student and telling him he needed to crave wisdom like he craved air while held underwater. Businessmen are instructed to crave sales in this way.

Sadly, Hittleman's scientifically unsound beliefs on healthy living weren't enough to save him from dying from cancer in his mid-sixties, with Ami Chen Mills reporting that 'According to friends, Richard's illness was an embarrassment to him, and hidden even from them.'[19] On the bright side – for Hittleman, at least – he managed to dodge the massive tax bill he'd built up by falsely claiming religious exemptions, instead leaving that bombshell for the wife he'd divorced to deal with.[20]

Hittleman was clearly on the make, deploying a tried-and-trusted cod-spirituality to nurture a cult-like devotion ripe for monetisation. With his faith-based approach to grifting, Hittleman now looks like a forerunner to far-right prosperity gospel megachurches such as Awaken in San Diego, whose pastor Jurgen Matthesius laces his sermons with vaccine denialism and QAnon-style attacks on election fraud and global cabals. His flock are expected to tithe 10 per cent of their income so that God can bless them with health and wealth, and to give generously regardless of their means and even if they can't afford to, in order to be saved.[21] Despite the creationist beliefs Hittleman shares with right-wing evangelicals, the wisdom dispensed in his published books on yoga appears positively restrained compared to the writing of Frank Rudolph Young, to whom we now turn.

13
Pull the Wool Over Your Own Eyes with Frank Rudolph Young, the 'Einstein' of Occult Yoga

While Richard Hittleman represents the 'faith-based' version of postural practice, Frank Rudolph Young can be seen as the epitome of those pedalling a more pseudo-scientific, occult vision of modern yoga. It is instructive to home in on these two figures, as most contemporary yoga practitioners seem to fall somewhere between the two poles. In terms of the yoga trajectory followed by Young, Aleister Crowley and Felix Guyot loom large, with universal occult 'truth' favoured over the 'local' colour of Hindu religious rites and beliefs.

In his tome *Psychic City Chicago*, Brad Steiger says:

> Although I have never met Frank Rudolph Young in person, I don't know anyone who has either! ... But this mysterious Chicago recluse, who is known in certain esoteric circles as the 'Einstein of the Occult,' intrigues me so much that I have been compelled to interview him as best I could [via correspondence].[1]

Steiger isn't the only person supposed 'yoga expert' Young has intrigued, with the lack of solid biographical information doing nothing to damp down the swell of underground interest that has risen over the past two decades in both physical culture and occultist circles.[2]

As far as can be determined, Frank Rudolph Young was born on 16 April 1911 in Panama City. At the age of 17 he moved to the United States, arriving in New York City on 17 September 1928 on the *Santa Teresa* passenger ship. Young informed Brad Steiger in his correspondence interview that 'Aside from my ancestral background, I had been researching the occult from a mere boy, right in the midst of the Voodoo center in the Republic of Panama, where I had been born of a Scotch-Irish mother and of an English-Spanish-East Indian father.'[3] Young appears to have died in Chicago in 2002 at the age of 91. While this might be regarded as a ripe old age, it fell somewhat short of his own (pseudo-scientific) expectations. In *The Yogatronic Diet*, Young asserts:

> In my long interview with Jeff Lyon for his 'Close Up' column ... I announced that I expect to live to 330 years old or longer. Nearly a million readers considered that ridiculous. A week later, however, the *Los Angeles Times* reported that Russian scientists believed that human beings could not only live 100 years but up to 400 years longer.[4]

An in-part factually questionable page by Greg Joel Newton on the now defunct *Lionquest Fitness* website was for a decade or so the go-to repository for online information about Young, including an unsubstantiated claim that he authored the Mike Marvel Dynaflex muscle-building course:

> Young was a doctor of chiropractic medicine and occultist who practiced something called 'Zohar' science. He cultivated an air of mystery about himself ... Supposedly he was descended from a long line of Indian Yogis ... I was contacted one time by a man who said he knew Dr. Young

> personally. According to him ... Young was very private, secretive, and paranoid ... So why is there a page devoted to Dr. Young? For one thing, the Dynaflex course and the Sinkram courses are remarkably simple, but effective ways to train the muscles without tearing the body down ... Young also grasped the concept that the various glands of the body were stimulated by various body movements and tensing he called 'asanas.' However, he also tied these things to occult practices and necromancy.[5]

Like many yogis and old school strongmen, Young was clearly steeped in New Thought. On top of stressing positive thinking and self-belief, however, he often seeks to achieve health and physical rejuvenation through bodily realignment. As a result, his occult beliefs are often inseparable from his yoga and physical culture teachings. To give a taste of Young's leanings with regard to the former, he promised readers of his most popular occult book, *Cyclomancy*, that they could obtain a number of 'powers' should they follow the instructions provided. These include the power to 'travel with your astral body', 'see into the future with a crystal ball' and 'stay slim without starvation'.[6]

Constructing a full bibliography of Young's work is not easy. Young became obsessed with proving he'd discovered various health and psychic 'truths' years before anyone else, but when referring back to his earlier work would provide references that didn't include the pseudonyms he had originally used. For example, in *Yoga Secrets of Extraordinary Health & Long Life*, Young cites a book he wrote called *Solar Diet*, but doesn't explain that it was published under the name Rex Grant.[7] Similarly, Young made copyright registrations for books and pamphlets in both his own name and a variety of alternatives, including Maranedi El Krishnar, Zohar Science, Zohar School, Gaucho, and – as just noted – Rex Grant.[8] From the early 1950s onwards, Young penned a stream of mail order works on self-improvement through physical culture, as well as the related areas of self-defence, diet, occult 'development', 'correct' thinking and mental 'efficiency'.

By the time Young bagged a publishing contract with the mainstream operation Parker in the mid-1960s, he already had a wealth of material from his slew of self-development pamphlets, courses and books to draw and expand upon. Much of this writing over the prior decade had involved recycling the same material in different publications. For instance, the copyright page for 1953 publication *X-Ray Mind: A Krishnara Course* – written under the pen name Maravedi El Krishnar – indicates the publication is a compendium of two previous works: *Analyse People at Sight* (1952) and *X-Ray Mind* (1952, updated 1953).[9] In this publication, under the subheading 'KRISHNARA The Science of the Superman', Young asserts in somewhat sinister fashion:

KRISHNARA is not for the trifler or for the mere bookworm. It is for you if you aspire to become an all-around Superman or Superwoman, mentally, physically, socially and sexually. In X-RAY MIND, Krishnara trains you how to analyse people at sight and dominate them at will. In GRAN-SEXRON, it brings you the absolute power over the opposite sex. In MIRACLE MIND, it can mold your mind into a 'genius'.[10]

Young then spends a hundred pages talking about how to identify the 42 different personality types he claims to have categorised. Having made the identification, all the reader need do is follow Young's instructions on how to manipulate them. For example, when it comes to Miss Jelly Fish type: 'Flatter her without reservation. Despite her embarrassed smile, she falls heavily for flattery.'[11] There then follows a section on 'Dangerous Power: Develop A Yoga Like Mind' with exercises such as 'The Unconquerable Eye': 'This eye fits best a king, dictator, commander, executive and others with authority over others. Stare in the mirror into your own eyes and think of yourself as possessing incomparable mental power.'[12] The megalomania implied by these words seems a clear throwback to the attitudes of the pre-Second World War fascist yogis.

Shortly thereafter, we arrive at 'The Aloof Eye', which:

> ... enables you to engage in silent conversation with the object of your interest and stir up her emotions ... This effect is absolutely necessary for romance. Few women are thrilled by the man who does not arouse in them feelings of danger. Not brutal danger, but danger of their ruin.[13]

The underhand, manipulative misogyny apparent in Young's writing is a clear precursor to the methods employed by what's now known as the 'pickup artist', whose lineage can be traced back through works such as *How To Pick Up Girls* (1970) by Eric Weber and *The Art of Erotic Seduction* (1967) by Albert Ellis and Roger Conway.[14] Young, however, doesn't emphasise responsibility the way Ellis and Conway do. Instead, he offers techniques such as 'the call of Svengali' – one of several gimmicks that place him closer to the more cynical pickup artists of recent decades than the men often cited as their precursors. Like these contemporary pickup artists, Young encourages his followers to develop both their inner game (their self-esteem and understanding of psychology) and their outer game (physical fitness, health, longevity). Ultimately, the inner and the outer can't be separated in Young's eyes, as is clear from his description of 'The Masterful Gait' in *X-Ray Mind*: 'Masterful carriage, moreover, is as much a mental acquisition as a physical one. It alters your whole mental output; not only because you feel different, but because others react differently to you.'[15]

The final page of *X-Ray Mind* lists a number of other, already published titles, including *Gran-Sexron: Absolute Power Over the Opposite Sex* and *How To Be Popular and Successful in 24 Hours – Evil power used for good*. Other publications that were (as far as can be ascertained) issued over the course of the next couple of years or so range from the relatively innocuous (*How To Cure Smoking – With Psychic Power*) to the ludicrously overblown (*Satanism – Deadly Orgies and Insidious Powers Over Others*). The list is seemingly endless. Moving further ahead, in 1960, the copyrights Young registered appear to be entirely physical culture orientated, such as a series of 'Big Muscles the Quick Way' pamphlets.

Young's first book issued by a mainstream publishing house (Parker) was *The Laws Of Mental Domination*,[16] which, as the Introduction makes clear, is very much a continuation of his mail order courses of the early and mid-1950s: 'By the end of the *Second Law* you will already be commanding others with your THOUGHTS. By the end of the *Fourth Law* you will be holding people – even PERFECT STRANGERS – spellbound at a glance.'[17]

Young's next book for Parker, *Cyclomancy*, continues in the same vein of repackaging material previously sold as mail order courses. In doing so, it contains some telling sentences about the self-delusion necessary to actually use the book as a 'self-help' manual:

You cannot expect to rule the rest of your body, much less the minds and bodies of others, with psychic power commands unless you can rule your own mind with them first. Exercise 1 brings you that power – the power to compel your own logical, reasoning conscious mind to accept the very opposite of what it knows to be true by just sending it a psychic power command from your Psychic Power Centre.[18]

Echoing Felix Guyot's mind control exercises discussed previously, this exercise consists of putting your left hand in a bowl of cold water and convincing yourself the water is very warm.

Although *Cyclomancy* is one of Young's mind power books, 'Lesson 7' – entitled 'How Never To Get Tired By Putting Your Muscle Tone Under Psychic Power Control' – is essentially a 15-page chapter on physical exercise, including workout instructions. In fact, each of Young's books feature variations on very repetitive exercises. In 1967's *The Secrets Of Personal Psychic Power*, for instance, there are various versions of staring at yourself in a mirror, then transforming your perceived reflection into the likeness of the person you wish to influence and mentally hurling a thought picture into the 'psychic power centre', which is allegedly located in your target's forehead.[19]

Alongside the exercises to develop psychic power, *Secrets Of Personal Psychic Power* also contains case studies of individuals who have allegedly benefited from the techniques.[20] This provides a convenient means of padding the book to its required commercial length. The case studies are, however, about as believable as the sketch of Young provided in the Introduction, in which this recluse grandiosely claims that he:

> ... and his two great-granduncles, his grandfather and father, spent a total of 131 years searching the continents of the world for the well guarded secrets of psychic power ... During 35 of those years, Frank R. Young himself *met, studied under, knew* or *associated* with ex-President Herbert Hoover, billionaire Bernard Baruch, immortal authors and artists like Ernest Hemingway, Sinclair Lewis, Thomas Wolfe; exciting religious leaders like Aimee Semple

McPherson, and Krishna Venta; Dr. Eisenschim; Dr. Sadler, the noted psychiatrist and textbook author; many renowned university professors; a galaxy of Hollywood stars; and many other kinds of successful people in different professions.[21]

There was more of the same in 1968's *Psychastra*, which claimed the Young family's psychic search had in fact lasted 'over 140 years'.[22] Thus, with the stroke of a pen, nine more years had been added to his family's epic quest for occult knowledge. A year later, *Yoga For Men Only* was published. The Christian cultural basis – rerun via New Thought – of Young's outlook can be seen in his repeated use of the phrase the 'four horsemen of the mastabah', which invokes the biblical 'four horsemen of the apocalypse' but substitutes the last word for a term denoting a type of ancient Egyptian tomb. The yoga course Young offers men is intended to help them overcome these four horsemen, which he flags as the down pull of gravity, faulty posture, weight-bearing, and ground resistance.[23] Many of the exercises are rooted in isometrics but instead of the more usual single seven-second hold, two seconds is recommended with repetitions.

The 'case studies' provided of how Young's yoga system has transformed lives are revealing of his attitude to women, even if their veracity is somewhat in doubt. Take the example of 'Harry':

> In less than two weeks Harry had tightened up his loose waist noticeably ... Harry tackled Ava again on the extravagance question ... his new manly aggressiveness and driving capacity caught her unawares. *Within a couple of weeks Harry was the much cherished master of his home!*[24]

This is followed by an equally unlikely example of 'real life' transformation under the subheading: 'How rundown 58-year old Vincent won for himself a 32-year-old wife'.[25] While Young recommends some of his yogametrics exercises for mere physical fitness, others allegedly provide those who use them with the power of leadership. In fairness, such claims are no more ridiculous than run-of-the-mill yoga teachers proclaiming that their postural practice will lead to wisdom or spiritual growth. In places, Young actually offers sounder advice on exercise safety than many yoga teachers I've encountered, cautioning that 'Unless you are doing them under doctor's orders, avoid exercises that bend your spine backwards.'[26] Elsewhere, however, as in the self-defence section, *Yoga For Men Only* owes more to comic book mythology than practical research. To perform Young's 'yoga freeze', one must adopt the stance of a person ready to spring at their adversary and rip them apart, thereby deterring the opponent from attacking you. Similarly, the 'yoga rout' involves moving in ways that confuse and alarm a potential attacker, once again putting them off launching an assault.[27]

In the books Young wrote after *Yoga For Men Only*, he drew back slightly from his obsession with big muscles signifying power and providing mental strength, instead writing about how his exercises not only helped build muscles in men but assisted in 'slenderizing' women. This was a smart move, given that women formed a considerable proportion of the market for self-help books. Thus, with *Yoga Secrets For Extraordinary Health and Long Life*, Young pitched his words of wisdom at both men and women curious about yoga. As might be expected, the book is packed with the exaggerated claims and fictitious case studies the reader has come to expect from Young and his publisher Parker. This time the physical exercises are called '*mov-asanas*', and alongside the isometrics there are drills such as 'A Yogi's Daily Psychic Power Trigger'.

This particular exercise involves writing 'on a piece of paper the name of the person you want to win, or the goal you wish to achieve', before – among other steps – pressing 'your head down hard upon the paper' and driving 'the full power of your nerve-electricity into it'.[28]

Further ratcheting up the absurdity of *Yoga Secrets* is such eye-opening sex-related advice as:

> Your pubic hair, whether you are a man or a woman, multiplies genital heat (crotch or pelvic heat). The multiplied heat can overexcite the sex glands because it penetrates deep into their adjoining tissues. It can convert a controlled individual into a sexual-activity slave or a masturbation addict, draining off nerve-electricity. To protect yourself against this wasteful sapping of your physical voltage shave off your pubic hair once a month! ... as a sex aid for a man, shaving off pubic hairs permits the sex organ to enlarge more during sexual intercourse. This is because no significant amount of crotch heat is drained off into his mate through interlocking pelvic hairs ... Yogis who rejoined the material world have maintained erections for eight hours of rather continuous copulation.[29]

When Young published this passage in the 1970s, having a big bush was fashionable both in the general population and pornography, so asking readers to shave off their public hair went against the mainstream grain in a way it doesn't now. Presumably it was a small price to pay for eight hours of sex.

Several of the exercises featured in Young's books are also regularly taught in present-day gym yoga classes. That said, Young likes to push things to the next level, so while many yoga lessons end with a few minutes of corpse pose, in *Cyclomancy* 'the Einstein of the Occult' advises readers to lie in what he calls 'dead man' position for 30 minutes, twice a day.[30]

Young followed *Yoga Secrets For Extraordinary Health* with *Zodiac Force Control*, a more overtly mystical tome that begins in typical megalomaniac fashion: 'I, Frank Young, appear to be the only person ever known to possess the Evolving Kundalini Eye (THE EKE). This astounding mystic eye is perceived even more readily in my photograph on the back of this book than in person.'[31] The mentioned photo is the same one used in his *X-Ray Mind* course in the early 1950s. The book features a breathing technique designed to draw '*odic* force' into the body, as well as instructions on how to project this force for the purposes of healing.[32] Later, the book explains how to perform psychic surgery,[33] which features a pre-emptive rant about why the technique is not – repeat *not* – a hoax:

> The purpose of this book is to teach you the technique of psychic healing, not to fill the pages proving it. If you don't believe it works, it might never work for you. If you strongly believe in it, though, you can develop into a miracle healer.[34]

In other words, if Young's techniques don't work for you, then you only have yourself to blame – which is convenient for the author, but something of a let-down for the reader.

Young's final book for a mainstream publisher – at least under his legal name – was *The Yogatronic Diet*.[35] Young himself acknowledges this is a repackaging of his earlier work, *Solar Diet*:

> In the 24 years following the publishing of *Solar Diet*, I have leaped another 24 years ahead of present-day science. With the *Yogatronic Diet*, I have expanded *Solar Diet* to six times its length and have added to it the miracle-making Triple Tonic Secret.[36]

Length-wise, this appears to be hyperbole given that Google Books lists *Solar Diet* as being 140 pages long, while *The Yogatronic Diet* comes in at a not particularly weighty 244 pages. Moreover, the later book is once again padded out with unsubstantiated 'case studies', which calls into question how much new information there actually is. When it comes to dietary advice, the previously mentioned '*odic* force' makes another appearance. 'The *odic force* is an emanation present in every substance, living or dead ... It was discovered by Baron von Reichenbach in 1848 ... You can extract the utmost nutrition out of every food you eat, through its odic force.'[37]

The occult cranks extolling *odic* force – or *od* to use Reichenbach's broad term for what he claimed to be investigating – often admit that it resembles the Indian concept of *prana*, Chinese notions of *chi* or *qi*, and Japanese *ki*. That said, rather than being a universal occult truth, *odic* force is the product of vitalist pseudo-science. As Martin Gardner observes in *Fads and Fallacies in the Name of Science*:

> The history of modern physics is spotted with reports of nonexistent radiations, and it is not unusual for the discoverer to attribute dowsing and similar occult phenomena to them. A good example is the nineteenth century discovery of a force called 'Od' by German physicist Baron Karl von Reichenbach.[38]

What useful advice there is in *The Yogatronic Diet* can be summed up as follows: eat clean (i.e., don't eat processed foods), eat three meals a day and don't snack; get sufficient sleep; don't drink alcohol or smoke tobacco, and exercise. As the reader may glean, none of this advice is revolutionary. The remainder of the book is largely impenetrable waffle and filler, including Young's much repeated hogwash about living to be over 300 years old. The following gives a flavour of what is on offer:

> I urge you, hereafter, to fall in love with your own waist, the axis of your whole body! Turn physiologically narcissistic! Embrace total health and long-lasting youth as your constant mistress or lover! Explode with ecstasy from your waistline and ring with muscle tone! Cast out flabby relaxation from your whole body, and the negativity of mental suppression.[39]

And so it goes on. In his cranky peculiarity, Young is typical of many people attracted to both yogic spirituality and occultism more generally. Above all, in cultivating his deluded beliefs, he adopts a pick-and-mix approach to world culture. Starting from a culturally Christian base, his writing proceeds to sprinkle on elements from across the globe: a bit of Chinese ying and yang here, some Hindu beliefs there, native practices from Central America elsewhere. Having done so, Young stirs in plenty of European occultism and dollops of supposedly 'scientific' information culled from academic papers and newspaper reports. The result is unadulterated bullshit rather than ancient wisdom. Nonetheless, Young's influence bubbles on through underground cliques, occasionally bursting out into the mainstream. For instance, in Edward Zwick's Hollywood movie *Love And Other Drugs* (2010), one of the characters — who might be described as a gullible and sexually frustrated pickup artist — is briefly shown reading a copy of Young's *The Secrets Of Personal Psychic Power*.

There have been two main strands to Young's fanbase in recent decades. Firstly, there are the true believers in the occult, who imagine they can achieve some of the powers described in Young's books — despite the fact he clearly didn't possess them himself — by following his instructions on 'psychic development'.[40] Secondly, he has enduring cult appeal among certain people interested in isometric/yoga exercises. From what I've encountered of this, these admirers are very often Christian, and while they claim to separate Young's physical culture teachings from what they see as his spirit conjurations, the impression given is that they're attracted to him precisely because he offers them a walk on the dark side.

What can the rest of us take from Young? Beyond lessons in how a con-artist operates and providing an example of the type of person who wishes to project the image of being an accomplished yogi, I would argue Young is an exemplar of the fusion of hucksterism and reactionary politics that has come to characterise much of modern postural practice, starting in the early twentieth century and continuing all the way up to the present day. Moreover, Young – perhaps more than any other Western yogi from the era in which he was active – can be seen as a precursor to the incels and pickup artists who make up a sizeable chunk of today's alt-right. The type of toxic masculinity spread by 'manosphere' influencers such as proud misogynist Andrew Tate, who hit the headlines after being charged with human trafficking, can be found pretty much fully formed in Young's mail order courses of the 1950s. In this respect, Tate's Hustler's University – essentially, a glorified online chat room offering get-rich-quick schemes based on cryptocurrency, copywriting and e-commerce, alongside tips on how men should handle women – bears a remarkable resemblance to Young's 1950s courses. Like Young, Tate is basically selling 'secret knowledge' that is based in a self-centred, cynical vision of the world, drawing on martial arts, health and fitness as a means of doing so.[41]

Conclusion

I concluded my historical account of modern postural practice in the 1970s for a number of reasons. After this date, both technological change and the growth in numbers of those practicing modern yoga meant no successor was able to match the fame and influence Richard Hittleman attained within modern postural practice via his TV programmes. With the spread of home video equipment and the proliferation of cable television in the 1980s, the ways in which home workouts were marketed tilted away from books and mail order courses. The audience for exercise materials in these new formats also continued to fragment. While there doesn't seem to have been much change in the form of physical postural practice classes, over the course of the decade remembered for the AIDS epidemic and the debut of MTV, the most fashionable workouts were branded as aerobics.

The expansion and development of the internet brought further changes, mostly after the turn of the millennium. Despite niche marketing within modern postural practice and an increasing proliferation of both styles and brands, it was with the internet that modern yoga, along with its evil twin the alt-right, rose to their current prominence. Nonetheless, what I've covered laid the ground for yoga as it is now. I've provided an account of the key figures that shaped modern postural practice as it exists today in many – particularly English-speaking – parts of the overdeveloped world. Most of those I encountered through yoga classes had only the vaguest notions, if any at all, of the actual – as opposed to mythological – history of what they practiced.

Although I did occasionally leave the London Borough of Islington to learn more about modern yoga, I didn't really need to do so. What was happening globally within modern postural practice was reflected locally. While I found the plastic mysticism of gym yoga classes ridiculous and annoying, some of the instructors would try to up the hippie-dippie ante by encouraging their students to find a 'deeper spirituality' beyond the gym. A couple of leisure centre postural practice teachers were pleased as punch when Tara Yoga opened in Ironmonger Row, pretty much next door to where they taught. There is now a BBC Radio 4 series about one woman's claims that within two years of joining that particular yoga centre she'd been sucked into a cult and was sexually trafficked.[1]

This and other Tara Yoga centres are linked to the teachings of Romanian 'guru' and convicted sex offender Gregorian Bivolaru. The BBC series *Bad Guru* is just the latest negative media coverage of Bivolaru and the Movement for Spiritual Integration into the Absolute he founded in 1990. Following ongoing legal issues in Romania, Bivolaru was granted asylum in Sweden after claiming that he had suffered religious persecution. In 2013, a Romanian court sentenced him to jail in absentia. Three years later he was arrested in Paris and extradited, before fleeing Romania in 2017.[2] In November 2023, Bivolaru was arrested again in France on charges of organised kidnap, rape and abuse.[3]

The gym instructors who recommended the Tara Yoga centre had apparently attended some classes there and were impressed by them. It wasn't the first questionable recommendation they'd made. One of them repeatedly suggested that their students try attending the North London Buddhist Centre for meditation. This Buddhist Centre was part of the Triratna organisation and I'd first heard about its culture of sexual abuse decades earlier when it was known as the Friends of the Western Buddhist Order. The press didn't get on the case of this duplicitous cult until some years after this.[4] Since I had no desire to meditate and wouldn't have gone near Triratna even if you paid me, I was in no danger from these recommendations, but I wasn't the only person hearing them. While none of the instructors I encountered at my local gym showed any sign of being interested in politics, there were students who made no secret of the far-right culture war ideologies they embraced.

I permanently knocked any form of yoga practice on the head in 2019, and at the same time switched all my other workouts to home training. So I wasn't around to hear the anti-vax, anti-mask rhetoric spread in modern postural practice classes about the measures designed to mitigate the Covid pandemic. That said, it wasn't unusual to hear anti-vax and anti-Big Pharma rhetoric before or after the gym yoga sessions I did attend. This was when anti-vax delusions were centred on MMR,[5] and before ritual denunciations of Big Pharma started to get wrapped up into transphobic rants about puberty blockers. Those of us who value our HIV+ friends whose lives were saved by 'Big Pharma' tend to have more nuanced views of these subjects.

I saw claims online and from around the world about Covid I was pleased not to have to endure in person from new age yogis. One of many instances that caught my eye was Australian yoga studio Egg Of The Universe comparing fully vaxed freedoms to segregation.[6] This was memorable because of the stereotypical way it hijacked progressive discourse for a reactionary cause. I wasn't surprised to see further newspaper headlines about Sydney's Egg Of The Universe a few years down the line, this time for trading while insolvent and failing to pay superannuation and wages, while at the same time the company that owned the yoga studio made generous loans to its founders.[7]

Moving on, my overriding hope is the story told in this book will discourage those thinking of taking up modern postural practice for health reasons from doing so – they can more effectively pursue other forms of exercise for this end. That said, I can't and wouldn't want to prohibit modern yoga. Nevertheless, if someone wishes to pursue a back-bending yoga practice – or become a contortionist – they should know in advance that it may result in long-term physical injuries. Likewise, they should be aware that most of the claims made about modern postural practice are at best hype, and for the most part mythological.

Given the sheer amount of yoga fakery out there, it is entirely possible that the real origins of modern postural practice may never be known with anything approaching absolute certainty. Even so, the fabrication of false guru lineages by many of the leading figures of modern yoga is now well documented. In light of this widespread trickery, it seems clear enough that the exercise systems propounded by these figures do not have any kind of ancient provenance.

Finally, while the batshit-insane beliefs and proclamations of the historical figures examined in this book might provide us all with hours of amusement, they also give important insight into the techniques of the fascist yogis and new age hucksters of today, from QAnon yoga moms to snake-oil conspiracists such as the financially and morally bankrupt 'journalist' Alex Jones.

Notes

Introduction

1. Bill Hopkins was repeatedly named in Italian court proceedings as a key London contact of the far-right terrorists responsible for the Bologna Station bombing and other atrocities: 'A Tangled Web Of Fascists, Fugitives And Secret Ops' by Alfio Bernabei, *Searchlight Magazine*, Spring 2022, 16–17.
2. See 'Scandal Contorts Future Of John Friend, Anusara Yoga' by Manuel Roig-Franzia, *Washington Post*, 28 March 2012.
3. *Anusara Yoga Teacher Training Manual* by John Friend, Anusara Press, Texas, 2005, updated seventh edition.
4. 'HBO's Breath Of Fire Explores The Sudden Fall Of Celebrity Yoga Teacher Guru Jagat' by Oliva B. Waxman, *Time Magazine*, 23 October 2024.
5. See, for example, *The Triumph of the Moon: A History of Modern Pagan Witchcraft* by Ronald Hutton, Oxford University Press, 1999.
6. See *Yoga In Practice* edited by David Gordon White, Princeton University Press, Princeton, NJ 2012, 2. In recent years, there has been a strand of academic yoga research that places emphasis on the origins of modern postural yoga lying in Western gymnastics and European bodybuilding. The best-known work ploughing this field is *Yoga Body: The Origins of Modern Posture Practice* by Mark Singleton. One of the many texts that paved the way for Singleton's book was *A History of Modern Yoga: Patanjali and Western Esotericism* by Elizabeth De Michelis, in which the author observes: 'English, by the way, can be stated to be the language of Modern Yoga. This is a clear indication of its cultural roots': *Yoga Body: The Origins of Modern Posture Practice* by Mark Singleton, Oxford University Press, 2010; *A History of Modern Yoga: Patanjali and Western Esotericism* by Elizabeth De Michelis, Continuum, London and New York 2004, 8 footnote.

7. '"Call Me A Racist, But Don't Say I'm A Buddhist": Meet America's alt right. They present themselves as modern thinkers of extremism. But the US far right, discovers Sanjiv Bhattacharya, have the same white supremacist obsessions' by Sanjiv Bhattacharya, *The Observer*, 9 October 2016.
8. *People: Eric Atwood, 41, Of Manhattan Beach CA: Avowed Neo-Nazi & 'Unite The Right' Attendee* by Pacific Antifascist Research Collective, 28 February 2022. Last accessed 14 November 2024: https://web.archive.org/web/20240425051434/https://pacantifa.is/people/eric-lyle-atwood-manhattan-beach-nazi/
9. *Neo-Nazi Terrorism and Countercultural Fascism: The Origins and Afterlife of James Mason's Siege* by Spencer Sunshine, Routledge, Oxfordshire 2024, see Part IV.
10. 'Active Club Network' by Anti-Defamation League, *ADL* website. Last accessed 25 November 2024: https://web.archive.org/web/20241113072824/https://www.adl.org/resources/backgrounder/active-club-network
11. *Conspirituality: How New Age Conspiracy Theories Became A Health Threat* by Derek Beres, Matthew Remski and Julian Walker, Public Affairs, New York 2023.
12. *Practice And All Is Coming: Abuse, Cult Dynamics And Healing In Yoga And Beyond* by Matthew Remski, Embodied Wisdom Publishing, Rangiora 2019, 92.
13. 'Why You Should Know About The New Thought Movement' by Christopher H. Evans, *The Conversation*, 15 February 2017. Last accessed 27 October 2024: http://web.archive.org/web/20241007165918/https://theconversation.com/why-you-should-know-about-the-new-thought-movement-72256
14. 'Covid Free' by Marco Mandrino, *Hari-Om* blog, 9 June 2021. Last accessed 14 November 2024: https://archive.ph/RgyAj
15. 'Does anyone remember, according to ancient tradition, what Yoga is for?' by Marco Mandrino, *Hari-Om* blog, 3 February 2023. Last accessed 14 November 2024: https://archive.ph/BSTVs
16. 'That Religion Called Science' by Marco Mandrino, *Hari-Om* blog, 31 July 2023. Last accessed 14 November 2024: https://archive.ph/PDvOi
17. 'I Have What I Have Given (G. D'Annunzio)' by Marco Mandrino, *Hari-Om* blog, 3 January 2023. Last accessed 14 November 2024: https://archive.ph/ZEGwl

18. 'R@c?sm and awareness' by Marco Mandrino, *Hari-Om* blog, 15 April 2024. Last accessed 14 November 2024: https://archive.ph/8L1zb

Part I
Happy Baby: A Grubby Guru Takes Us All to the Cleaners

1. '*Rolling Stone* Will Replace Top Editor' by David Carr, *New York Times*, 29 April 2002, Section C1.

1   Did Pierre Bernard Invent Yoga in California at the Start of the Twentieth Century?

1. See, for example, *The Path of Modern Yoga: The History of an Embodied Spiritual Practice* by Elliott Goldberg, Inner Traditions, Rochester, VT, 2016.
2. Singleton, *Yoga Body*.
3. *The Great Oom: The Improbable Birth of Yoga in America* by Robert Love, Viking, New York 2010, 9.
4. Love, *The Great Oom*, 350 (Notes).
5. 'The Omnipotent Oom: Tantra and Its Impact on Modern Western Esotericism' by Hugh B. Urban, *Esoterica: Journal of Esoteric Studies* 3, 2001, 218–239.
6. Love, *The Great Oom*, 12–13.
7. Love, *The Great Oom*, 154.
8. Love, *The Great Oom*, 350–351. This is where the guru lineage claims for Hamati are located.
9. This is listed in Love's index as *Vira Sadhana: International Journal of the Tantrick Order*. The issue is numbered Vol. 5, No. 1 but appears to be the first and only edition of the journal.
10. *International Journal: Tantrik Order*, 94–95.
11. Love, *The Great Oom*, 33.
12. Love, *The Great Oom*, 20.
13. *The Subtle Body: The Story of Yoga In America* by Stefanie Syman, Farrar, Straus & Giroux, New York 2010, 313, 'Notes to pages 80–85'.

14. *Theos Bernard, The White Lama: Tibet, Yoga, and American Religious Life* by Paul G. Hackett, Columbia University Press, New York 2012, 431.
15. 'Remembering Ourselves: On Some Countercultural Echoes of Contemporary Tantric Studies' by Jeffrey J. Kripal, *Religions of South Asia*. 1 (1): 28 November, 2007. Last accessed 27 November 2023, archived online here: https://web.archive.org/web/20190417175425/http://danbhai.com/anthro_of_hinduism/RememberingOurselves.pdf
16. Urban, 'The Omnipotent Oom'.
17. Coué was a French psychologist famous for his affirmation 'Each day, in every way, I am getting better and better.'
18. Syman, *The Subtle Body*, 111.
19. Love, *The Great Oom*, 82.

2 The Great Oom and White Power

1. 'Yoga in America: History, Community Formation, and Consumerism' by Rebecca Anne D'Orsogna, University of Texas at Austin 2013. Published in book form under the same title by Lawchakra on 25 February 2023, ISBN-13 9781805242284.
2. Love, *The Great Oom*, 245.
3. *Eastern Philosophy For Western Minds* by Hamish McLaurin, The Stratford Company, Boston, MA 1933, 3–6.
4. McLaurin, *Eastern Philosophy For Western Minds*, 13–15.
5. D'Orsogna, 'Yoga in America', 2013, 128.
6. *International Journal: Tantrik Order*.
7. D'Orsogna, 'Yoga in America', 2013, 104–105. The attraction of Diana and Viola Wertheim to Oom via his unsavoury media reputation is also covered here.

Part II
Warrior One, Two and Three: Fascism + Yoga = Fascist Yoga (The 1920s to the 1940s)

1. *Hatha Yoga* by Yogi Ramacharaka, Yogi Publishing Society, Chicago, IL 1904. UK edition by L. N. Fowler, London circa 1904, 203–1904.

2. *The Celestial Tradition: A Study of Ezra Pound's The Cantos* by Demetres P. Tryphonopoulos, Wilfrid Laurier University Press, Ontario 1992, 65–67 and 94, footnote 10.
3. John Kasper (1929–98) was a suspect in a school bombing in Nashville as well as a number of synagogue bombings. See John Kasper's FBI files obtained through the FOIA and hosted at the Internet Archive. Last accessed 18 September 2023; this is the first of them: https://archive.org/details/foia_Kasper_John-HQ-1
4. *John Kasper and Ezra Pound: Saving the Republic* by Alec Marsh, Bloomsbury, London 2015, 48–49.
5. *Smile Or Die: How Positive Thinking Fooled America & The World* by Barbara Ehrenreich, Granta Books, London 2009, 79–96.
6. *India and the Occult: The Influence of South Asian Spirituality on Modern Western Occultism* by Gordan Djurdjevic, Palgrave Macmillan, London 2014, 38.
7. *Book 4* first published in *The Equinox*, Vol. I, No. VIII, London 1912.
8. *Eight Lectures*, Yoga For Yahoos Lesson 2, Point 4. Last accessed 3 January 2024, archived here: https://web.archive.org/web/20201101052409/https://enfolding.org/yoga-magic-and-deception-iv/
9. 'Sri Sabhapati Swami and the "Translocalization" of Śivarājayoga', by Keith Cantú, UC Santa Barbara PhD, 2021, 448. Last accessed 3 January 2024, online here: https://escholarship.org/content/qt48v5t1bc/qt48v5t1bc.pdf
10. Among his (D'Annunzio's) close collaborators in Fiume was Guido Keller: a bisexual, naturist, Dadaist, yoga-practising wild man, who, like D'Annunzio, had a passion for daredevil flights, and whose role in Fiume was to organise pirate raids to replenish the always depleted supplies in the city': 'The Fascist Precursor' by Aidan O'Malley, *Dublin Review Of Books*, May 2021. Last accessed 27 November 2024: https://web.archive.org/web/20240225085458/https://drb.ie/articles/the-fascist-precursor/

3 Guido Keller and the Rijeka Yoga Group

1. *The Birth of Fascist Ideology* by Zeev Sternhell, Princeton University Press, Princeton, NJ 1989.

2. *The First Duce: d'Annunzio at Fiume* by Michael A. Ledeen, Transaction Publishers, New Brunswick, NJ, 3rd edition 2009, xiii for John The Baptist of fascism; 'How Rijeka Became The World's First Fascist State' by Jonathan Bousfield, *Time Out*, n.d. circa 2019 for cocaine, etc. Last accessed 28 November 2024: https://web.archive.org/web/20190930205608/https://www.timeout.com/croatia/things-to-do/how-rijeka-became-the-worlds-first-facist-state
3. Ledeen, *The First Duce*, xiii–xiv.
4. *Gabriele D'Annunzio: Defiant Archangel* by John Woodhouse, Oxford University Press 2001, 333.
5. Stories about Keller's use of his bi-plane to plunder supplies can be found in many unreliable sources. These include 'The Country That Ran On Cocaine And Yoga' by Ned Donovan, *Terra Nullius*, 15 April 2024. The amount of cocaine available during D'Annunzio's occupation appears massively exaggerated, while interest in yoga was restricted to a tiny group around Keller. Last accessed 28 November 2024: https://web.archive.org/web/20240417173236/https://www.terranullius.world/p/the-country-that-ran-on-cocaine-and
6. *Futurism and Politics: Between Anarchist Rebellion and Fascist Reaction, 1909–1944* by Günter Berghaus, Berghahn Books, Oxford 1995,137.
7. 'Guido Keller' by Anon., *Oblique*, n.d. Last accessed 28 November 2024: https://web.archive.org/web/20100126045604/http://www.oblique.it/manifesto_keller.html
8. 'Fiume under D'Annunzio: An Incubator of Evil' by Beach Combing, *Strange History*, 17 April 2014. Last accessed 1 September 2023: https://web.archive.org/web/20201108092956/http://www.strangehistory.net/2014/04/17/fiume-and-dannunzio-an-incubator-of-evil/
9. *Giovanni Comisso, Un provinciale in fuga* by Luigi Urettin Treviso, Istresco, 2009, 106: 'Genio della razza italica, pervertito dalle idee democratiche e borghesi delle "razze negative", inglesi, francesi e soprattutto ebrei.'
10. *Reading and Writing Italian Homosexuality: A Case of Possible Difference* by Derek Duncan, Ashgate, Aldershot 2006, 77.

11. *Seaport Of Love* by Janez Jansa and Domenico Quaranta, translated by Anna Carruthers, Aksioma, Institute for Contemporary Art, Ljubljana, Slovenia, 2009.
12. 'A City for Poets and Pirates' by Reinaldo Laddaga, *Cabinet*, Issue 58, Summer 2015.
13. O'Malley, 'The Fascist Precursor', *Dublin Review Of Books*, May 2021.
14. *Yoga. Sovversivi e rivoluzionari con d'Annunzio a Fiume* by Simonetta Bartolini, Luni Editrice, Milan 2019. Last accessed 29 November 2024: http://web.archive.org/web/20240622052509/https://www.lunieditrice.com/product/yoga-sovversivi-e-rivoluzionari-con-dannunzio-a-fiume-simonetta-bartolini/
15. 'Gabriele D'Annunzio And The Culture of Violence' by Jonathan Bousfield, *Stray Satellite*, n.d. circa 1919. Last accessed 29 November 2024: http://web.archive.org/web/20210725020347/https://straysatellite.com/fiume/
16. I do not want to send readers to active fascist propaganda operations so here is a page about Guido Keller from a defunct far-right site that has been preserved at the Internet Archive: 'Legacy Of Me Ne-Frego' by Hangman, *Noose: The Online Fascist Zine*, 5 August 2016. Last accessed 29 November 2024: http://web.archive.org/web/20170224025857/http://ropeculture.org/2016/08/05/legacy-of-me-ne-frego/

4 *Military Theorist Major J. F. C. Fuller, Whose Concept of Blitzkrieg Became Standard Practice in Nazi Warfare*

1. 'Fascist Yogis: Martial Bodies and Imperial Impotence' by Kate Imy in *Journal of British Studies*, Vol. 55, No. 2, April 2016, 320–343.
2. Imy, 'Fascist Yogis', 328.
3. *The Star in the West: A Critical Essay Upon the Works of Aleister Crowley* by Captain J. F. C. Fuller, Walter Scott Publishing Company, London 1907.
4. Fuller, *The Star in the West*, 290.
5. *The Equinox*, Vol. I, No. IV, privately published, London 1910, 284–290. Fuller used the pen name Sam Hardy.

6. 'Remembering The West Hampstead "Holy Man" and his Cult of Women' by Marianne Colloms and Dick Weindling, *Ham & High*, 23 March 2015.
7. *The Equinox*, Vol. I, No. IV, 41–196.
8. *Yoga: A Study of the Mystical Philosophy of the Brahmins and Buddhists* by J. F. C. Fuller, Rider, London 1925, vii–viii.
9. Fuller, *Yoga*, 138.
10. Fuller, *Yoga*, 53.
11. *Fascist Quarterly*, No. 1, London, January 1935.
12. Fuller, *Yoga*, 46.

5 Bengal Lancer and Hitler Aficionado Francis Yeats-Brown

1. *Bengal Lancer* by Francis Yeats-Brown, Gollancz, London 1930. Published in the US as *The Lives of a Bengal Lancer*, Viking Press 1930.
2. *Francis Yeats-Brown 1886–1944* by Evelyn Wrench, Eyre and Spottiswoode, London 1948, 85.
3. It was a close-knit family in every sense given Wrench married a cousin, as did Yeats-Brown the first time he got hitched.
4. Wrench, *Francis Yeats-Brown 1886–1944*, 25.
5. Imy, 'Fascist Yogis', 336–337.
6. *Caught By The Turks* by Francis Yeats-Brown, Arnold, London 1919.
7. *Lancer At Large* by Francis Yeats-Brown, Gollancz, London 1936.
8. *Yoga Explained* by Francis Yeats-Brown, Gollancz, London 1937.
9. *Golden Horn* by Francis Yeats-Brown, Gollancz, London 1932. Issued as *Bloody Years* by Viking in the US.
10. Imy, 'Fascist Yogis', 336.
11. Wrench's biography has Yeats-Brown working at *The Spectator* in London in 1928 when Love has him involved with Bernard's flying club. Yeats-Brown was not a pilot, and says so on page 11 of *Caught By The Turks:* 'Now I am not a pilot, and know little of machines.' Wrench confirms this on page 44 of his biography, Yeats-Brown was 'gazetted as an *observer* in the Royal Flying Corps ... His term of service ... was destined to be brief ...' (emphasis added).

NOTES

12. Love, *The Great Oom*, 255.
13. Wrench, *Francis Yeats-Brown 1886–1944*, 183–184.
14. Wrench, *Francis Yeats-Brown 1886–1944*, 176.
15. For an outline of Yeats-Brown's fascist ideology, see his contribution to *The Spectator Booklets 1: Parliament Or Dictatorship?* entitled 'Alternatives To Democracy: The Corporate State'.
16. *Dogs of War* by Francis Yeats-Brown, Peter Davis, London 1934.
17. *Cry Havoc!* by Beverley Nichols, Jonathan Cape, London 1933.
18. Yeats-Brown, *Dogs of War*, 221–223.
19. Wrench, *Francis Yeats-Brown 1886–1944*, 172–173, 208, 224, 283 (Appendix A).
20. See Wrench, *Francis Yeats-Brown 1886–1944*, 282.
21. Love, *The Great Oom*, 256–257. Love cites one example of the article being reprinted in the *Chester Times* of 25 April 1935.
22. Yeats-Brown, *Yoga Explained*, 25.
23. *Yogic Physical Culture Or The Secret Of Happiness* by Seetharaman Sundaram, Brahmacharya Publishing, Bangalore, 1928 or 1929. The copy I consulted had the title reversed as *The Secret of Happiness Or Yogic Physical Culture* by Yogacharya Sundaram of Bangalore, 8th edition revised, Yoga Publishing House, Coimbatore, 2000. The revised edition seems to have first appeared in 1971. The photographs in it appear to date from the late 1920s.
24. Sundaram. *The Secret of Happiness Or Yogic Physical Culture*, 8th edition, 103.
25. *Practical Yoga For Women* by Harvey Day, Pelham, London 1969, 156.
26. Yeats-Brown, *Yoga Explained*, 74–75.
27. There are studies showing that in the past Hindus did eat beef. See *The Myth of the Holy Cow* by Dwijendra Narayan Jha, Verso, London 2002.
28. Wrench, *Francis Yeats-Brown 1886–1944*, 228.

6 *Jakob Wilhelm Hauer and His Influence on the Architect of the Nazi Holocaust Heinrich Himmler*

1. '"Ve hav vays of making you relax": How SS recommended yoga to death camp guards as a good way to de-stress' by Allan Hall, *Daily*

Mail, 22 February 2012. Last accessed 30 November 2024: http://web.archive.org/web/20200813213900/https://www.dailymail.co.uk/news/article-2104365/How-SS-recommended-yoga-death-camp-guards-good-way-stress.html?ito=feeds-newsxml
2. *Yoga im Nationalsozialismus: Konzepte, Kontraste, Konsequenzen* by Mathias Tietke, Ludwig, Kiel, 2011.
3. *New Religions and the Nazis* by Karla Poewe, Routledge, Oxon 2006, 11–12
4. Poewe, *New Religions and the Nazis*, 31–32.
5. Poewe, *New Religions and the Nazis*, 118.
6. *The Yoga Tradition: Its History, Literature, Philosophy and Practice* by Georg Feuerstein, Hohm Press, Prescott, AZ, new edition 2001.
7. 'The Yoga Tradition' by Christopher Locke, *The Mystic Bourgeoisie*, 17 February 2006. Last accessed 6 September 2023: https://web.archive.org/web/20060322231044/http://mysticbourgeoisie.blogspot.com/2006/02/yoga-tradition.html
8. *The Essence of Yoga: A contribution to the Psychohistory of Indian Civilisation* by Georg Feuerstein, Rider, London 1974.
9. 'Interview with Georg Feuerstein', by Richard Rosen, 10 October 1997. An abridged version appeared in *Yoga Journal* but for discussion of Hauer, see the longer version published on Rosen's website circa 2015. Last accessed 6 September 2023: https://web.archive.org/web/20180827080346/http://www.richardrosenyoga.com/interview-with-georg-feuerstein-1997.html
10. 'Is Yoga Cultural Appropriation?' by Phillipa Beck, *Full Circle Yoga*, 4 December 2019. Last accessed 30 November 2024: http://web.archive.org/web/20240112052158/https://www.full-circle-yoga.ca/is-yoga-cultural-appropriation/
11. Beck links to a blog by Dave Romanelli entitled *Evil Yogis? The Ultimate Oxymoron* which attributes the information to the *Daily Mail:* 'The first yoga studio opened in Berlin in 1937. As reported in the *Daily Mail* ... .' Beck re-orders some of Romanelli's words but uses the first sentence quoted here verbatim. Although Romanelli refers via the *Mail* piece to Himmler, he doesn't make Beck's false claim that Hitler was interested in yoga. Last accessed 19 December 2024: https://web.archive.org/web/20170208172759/https://yeahdave.com/yoga-and-the-nazis/

NOTES

7 Mircea Eliade, Julius Evola, Savitri Devi – National Socialism as a Religion and the Yoga of Power

1. In *Vremea*, Bucharest, 31 March 1935. An English translation by Cologero – seemingly a pen name of Toni Ciopa – can be found on traditionalist/alt-right website *Gornahoor*.
2. *Against the Modern World: Traditionalism and the Secret Intellectual History of the Twentieth Century* by Mark Sedgwick, Oxford University Press, 2004, 115–116.
3. Sedgwick, *Against the Modern World*, 115.
4. Sedgwick, *Against the Modern World*, 114.
5. See Sedgwick, *Against the Modern World*, 110–112.
6. *Yoga: Immortality and Freedom* by Mircea Eliade translated by Willard R. Trask, Princeton University Press paperback edition, Princeton, NJ 1970. It is dedicated to Eliade's fascist 'teacher' Nae Ionescu.
7. 'Recommended Yogi Reading' by YJ Editors, *Yoga Journal*, last updated 2 September 2021. Last accessed 1 December 2024: http://web.archive.org/web/20241201203257/https://www.yogajournal.com/lifestyle/balance/recommended-yogi-reading/
8. Eliade, *Yoga: Immortality and Freedom*, index page 495 for Evola and page 498 for Hauer.
9. *The Yoga of Power: Tantra, Shakti, and the Secret Way* by Julius Evola, Inner Traditions, Rochester, VT 1992, 2.
10. Evola, *The Yoga of Power*, 9.
11. Evola, *The Yoga of Power*, 189–190.
12. *Hitler's Priestess: Savitri Devi, the Hindu-Aryan Myth, and Neo-Nazism* by Nicholas Goodrick-Clarke, New York University Press, New York 2000.
13. *The Lightning and the Sun* by Savitri Devi, self-published by Savitri Devi, Calcutta 1958.
14. *Black Sun: Aryan Cults, Esoteric Nazism, and the Politics of Identity* by Nicholas Goodrick-Clarke, New York University Press, New York 2002, 173, 176, 178, 189.
15. 'Why Some New Age Influencers Believe Trump Is A "Lightworker"' by Nicole Karlis, *Salon*, 4 March 2021. This piece quotes 'experts' repeating a number of false claims about the Nazis and the occult. Nevertheless, it stands as a useful record of

the framing of Trump within 'pastel' QAnon as a lightworker. Last accessed 13 December 2024: http://web.archive.org/web/20241005112349/https://www.salon.com/2021/03/04/why-some-new-age-influencers-believe-trump-is-a-lightworker/

16. 'Gary Smith On Manoeuvres' (27 September 2010) and 'Rock Against Communism: The Roots Of Sol Invictus' (3 October 2010) both by Strelnikov, *Who Makes The Nazis*. Last accessed 30 December 2024: http://web.archive.org/web/20241130225925/http://whomakesthenazis.blogspot.com/search?q=Above+The+Ruins

17. Discogs entry for *Cavalcare La Tigre – Julius Evola: Centenary*. Last accessed 30 November 2024: http://web.archive.org/web/20220721044332/https://www.discogs.com/release/241423-Various-Cavalcare-La-Tigre-Julius-Evola-Centenary

18. Discogs entry for 'Hitler As Kalki' by *Current 93*. Last accessed 30 November 2024: https://www.discogs.com/master/704235-Current-93-Hitler-As-Kalki

19. 'Men's Current 93 Shirt 1988 Vintage t Shirt Neofolk Band t-Shirts Reprint Black' by Yao Chen on Amazon UK website, not dated. Last accessed 1 December 2024: http://web.archive.org/web/20241201150922/https://www.amazon.co.uk/YAO-CHEN-Current-Vintage-t-Shirts/dp/B0DFT8TS42

20. 'A Response To Sean Ragon' by Valdinoci, *NYC Antifa* blog, 6 November 2014. Last accessed 1 December 2024: http://web.archive.org/web/20240317090759/https://nycantifa.wordpress.com/2014/11/06/a-response-to-sean-ragon/

21. 'Of Runes and Love', Sean Ragon interviewed by Charlie Looker, *YouTube*, 24 September 2023. Last accessed 1 December 2024 (from 1.07.00): https://www.youtube.com/live/XlFbVNUkc5M

22. 'Runic Yoga or Stadha' by Misty Harker, *Satori By M Harker* blog, n.d. circa 2013. Last accessed 1 December 2024: http://web.archive.org/web/20241201170258/https://satoribymharker.wordpress.com/general-education-2/life-long-wellness/yoga-ii/

23. *Rune Might: The Secret Practices of the German Rune Magicians* by Edred Thorsson, Inner Traditions, Rochester, VT 2019 (original edition published in 1989).

24. 'Miguel Serrano's Antisemitism and its Impact on the Twenty-First-Century Countercultural Rightists' by Gustavo Guzmán, *Analysis of Current Trends in Antisemitism*, Vol. 40, No. 1, January

2019. Last accessed 19 December 2024: http://web.archive.org/web/20240804041145/https://www.degruyter.com/document/doi/10.1515/actap-2019-0001/html

Part III
Downward Dog: Occult Madness and Yogic Televangelism (Modern Postural Practice in the Post-war Era)

1. *Yoga in Britain: Stretching Spirituality and Educating Yogis* by Suzanne Newcombe, Equinox, Sheffield, 2019, 9. I consulted a pdf version of the book available for download online. Last accessed 6 October 2023: https://oro.open.ac.uk/50520/3/Newcombe_Yoga%20in%20Britain.pdf
2. *The Goddess Pose: The Audacious Life of Indra Devi, The Woman Who Helped Bring Yoga To The West* by Michelle Goldberg, Corsair, London 2016 (first published by Alfred A. Knopf, New York 2015), 134.
3. 'Michael Volin (Swami Karmananda)' on *Ageless Yoga* website. Last accessed 14 December 2024: http://web.archive.org/web/20190228025219/https://www.agelessyoga.com.au/pdf/volin.pdf
4. 'Lockdowns And Face Masks Really Did Help To Control Covid-19', by Michael Le Page, *New Scientist*, 24 August 2023. Last accessed 15 December 2024: https://web.archive.org/web/20241202154829/https://www.newscientist.com/article/2388929-lockdowns-and-face-masks-really-did-help-to-control-covid-19/; '"*Pastel* QAnon," Where Pro-Trump Conspiracy Theories Meet New Age Spirituality' by Caitlin Dickson, *Yahoo News*, 21 October 2020. Last accessed 14 December 2024: https://www.yahoo.com/news/pastel-q-anon-where-pro-trump-conspiracy-theories-meet-new-age-spirituality-222152937.html
5. 'Meet Krystal Tini of My Soul Mat in West Hollywood' by Anon., *VoyageLA*, 9 September 2019. Last accessed 14 December 2024: http://web.archive.org/web/20240205191647/https://voyagela.com/interview/meet-krystal-tini-soul-mat-west-hollywood/

8 Paul Dukes, Francis Yeats-Brown (Again) and Theos Bernard, Spreading the Great Oom's Gospel in the Post-war Years

1. The photographic section of the book can be found between pages 128 and 129 of *The Unending Quest: Autobiographical Sketches* by Sir Paul Dukes, KBE, Cassell & Co., London 1950.
2. Newcombe, *Yoga In Britain*, 149.
3. Dukes, *Unending Quest*, 126.
4. Dukes, *Unending Quest*, 129–130.
5. Yeats-Brown, *Yoga Explained*, 164.
6. Yeats-Brown, *Yoga Explained*, plate between pages 132 and 133.
7. Yeats-Brown, *Yoga Explained*, 136 and 149.
8. *Yoga For The Western World* appears to have been privately published in a number of editions by the author and/or a yoga organisation he headed. The copy I consulted was *Yoga For The Western World* by Sir Paul Dukes attributed both to the organisation Students of Western Yoga (on title page) and as published privately by the author (on copyright page), fourth edition, revised and enlarged November 1958, reprinted March 1959, no place of publication given but printed by O'Loughlin Brothers, Sydney.
9. *White Lama: The Life of Tantric Yogi Theos Bernard, Tibet's Emissary to the New World* by Douglas Veenhof, Harmony Books, New York, 2011, 19–21.
10. 'Theos Bernard and the Early Days of Tantric Yoga in America' by Paul G. Hackett in *Yoga In Practice* edited by White, 354–355.
11. Veenhof, *White Lama*, 28.
12. *Theos Bernard, The White Lama: Tibet, Yoga & American Religious Life* by Paul G. Hackett, Columbia University Press, New York 2012, 9, 73, 124.
13. Love, *The Great Oom*, 34.
14. Love, *The Great Oom*, 353.
15. Hackett, *Theos Bernard, The White Lama*, 431.
16. Hackett, *Theos Bernard, The White Lama*, 461.
17. Newcombe, *Yoga In Britain*, 31. It should be noted that footnote 125 of *Yoga In Britain* makes clear that Newcombe was unable to find any sales figures for major mid-century UK yoga and occult publisher Thorsons, while Rider's records of pre-war sales of its

yoga books appear to have been lost when their London offices were destroyed by Nazi bombs during the Second World War. Also, while Newcombe draws attention to the editorial input of Gerald J. Yorke on *Yoga and Health* and *Light on Yoga*, he had no direct editorial involvement with Theos Bernard's book.

9 Indra Devi and Her Editors at Prentice Hall

1. Goldberg, *The Goddess Pose*, 185 and 271.
2. On Devi's first book for Prentice Hall, see Goldberg's *The Goddess Pose*, 170–175. See also *Forever Young, Forever Healthy* by Indra Devi, A. Thomas & Co, London 1955 (originally published by Prentice Hall 1953). For Devi's dedication 'to Sidney Field for helping me with the writing of this book', see unnumbered dedication page at front. For Devi on Ramacharaka, see page 3; for Devi on early connections to theosophy, see pages 4–5. For Devi on Krishnamacharya, see pages 18–21; for Devi on opening her studio in Hollywood, see page 22.
3. *Renew Your Life Through Yoga* by Indra Devi, Paperback Library, New York 1969 (first published by Prentice Hall 1963), 35. *Yoga: The Technique of Health and Happiness* by Eugenie Strakaty (Indra Devi's married name), Kitabistan, Allahabad, 1948.
4. Goldberg, *The Path of Modern Yoga*, 210.
5. Chapter 12 'The Strange Case of T. M. Krishnamacharya' in *The Yoga Sutra of Patanjali: A Biography* by David Gordon White, Princeton University Press, Princeton, NJ 2014, 197–224.
6. Goldberg, *The Path of Modern Yoga*, 95.
7. Devi, *Forever Young*, 81.
8. 'Magic Words' on *This American Life* hosted by Ira Glass, Chicago Public Media, originally aired 15 August 2014. Schaumberger's employer isn't identified but *Secrets From Beyond The Pyramids* and *The Magic Of Chantomatics* are identified as titles issued by the publisher he worked for. Both appeared under Prentice Hall imprint Parker Publishing. *Ultra-Psychonics: How to Work Miracles with the Limitless Power of Psycho-Atomic Energy*, credited to Walter Delaney (1975), was also published by Parker. Last accessed 13 December 2024: http://web.archive.org/web/20150211203417/

http://www.thisamericanlife.org/radio-archives/episode/532/transcript
9. Devi, *Forever Young*, 166–167.
10. The Armshaw speech is reproduced as 'Yoga And The Dowser' by J. Armshaw in *Prediction*, Vol. 32, No. 10, Croydon October 1966, 11, 12, 13 and 18. What I quote comes from page 12.
11. *Yoga For Americans: A Complete 6 Weeks' Course for Home Practice* by Indra Devi, Prentice Hall, Englewood Cliffs, NJ 1959.
12. *Yoga For You: A Complete 6 Weeks' Course for Home Practice* by Indra Devi, A. Thomas, Preston 1960.
13. Devi, *Yoga For Americans*, x.
14. Devi, *Yoga For Americans*, 37.
15. Goldberg, *The Path of Modern Yoga*, 106.
16. Devi, *Yoga For Americans*, 78.
17. Fuller quoted in Devi's *Yoga For Americans* on page 135 – the section on kundalini power begins on page 128.
18. Devi, *Yoga For Americans*, 147.

10 Harvey Day, a Hack Who Found Success with Books on Yoga

1. *Study And Practice Of Yoga* by Harvey Day, Thorsons, London 1953, 53–55; Devi, *Renew Your Life Through Yoga*, 163–171.
2. *Occult Illustrated Dictionary* by Harvey Day, Kaye & Ward Ltd, London 1975, inside back flap of dust jacket. More or less the same information can be found on the dust jacket of the *Encyclopaedia Of Natural Health and Healing* by Harvey Day, Kaye & Ward Ltd, London 1979.
3. *You, Too, Can Write For Money* by Harvey Day, A. Thomas, Preston 1961, 22–25.
4. *About Yoga: The Complete Philosophy* by Harvey Day, Thorsons, London 1951, 7.
5. Day, *About Yoga*, 9.
6. Day, *About Yoga*, 9.
7. Day, *About Yoga*, 14.
8. Day, *About Yoga*, 16.
9. Day, *The Study and Practice Of Yoga*, 8.

10. 'The Uncertain Spy', *BBC* website 9 February 2004. Last accessed 30 October 2023: https://web.archive.org/web/20040613054240/https://www.bbc.co.uk/insideout/yorkslincs/series5/iom_spy.shtml
11. Day, *About Yoga*, 18–19. *Yoga Illustrated Dictionary* by Harvey Day, Kaye and Ward, London 1971, 30. Day, *Occult Illustrated Dictionary*, 25.
12. The story appears in *Aleister Crowley, A Memoir of 666* by Alan Burnett-Rae, London, Victim Press, 1971. I found it in this retelling in 'Dr. Alexander Cannon: A Biographical Sketch of a Friend & Acquaintance of Aleister Crowley' on the *Red Flame* website. Last accessed 30 October 2023: https://web.archive.org/web/20040622171102/http://www.redflame93.com/Cannon.html
13. Day, *About Yoga*, 52.
14. Day, *About Yoga*, 36.
15. Day, *About Yoga*, 31 and 158; Day, *The Study And Practice Of Yoga*, 112–113.
16. Day, *About Yoga*, 42.
17. *The Hindu-Yogi Science Of Breath: A Complete Manual of the Oriental Breathing Philosophy of Physical, Mental, Psychic and Spiritual Development* by Yogi Ramacharaka, Yogic Publication Society, Chicago, IL 1903, and *Fourteen Lessons In Yogic Philosophy and Oriental Occultism* by Yogi Ramacharaka, Yogic Publication Society, Chicago, IL 1903: Day, *About Yoga*, 158.
18. Day, *About Yoga*, 90.
19. Day, *Study And Practice Of Yoga*, 7; Day, *About Yoga*, 158. *Yogic Home Exercises. Easy Course of Physical Culture for Men & Women* by Swarmi Sivananda, Taraporevala Sons & Co., Bombay 1944.
20. Day, *Study and Practice Of Yoga*, 53–55.
21. Day, *You, Too, Can Write For Money*, 124; original emphasis.
22. In *The Breath Of Life* by Harvey Day, Thorsons, London 1965, the bibliography on pages 125–126 even includes *Doctor From Lhasa* by the fake 'Tibetan monk' T. Lobsang Rampa – in reality, English plumber's son Cyril Henry Hoskin (1910–81). Despite Hoskin being exposed as a fraud in the late 1950s, Day describes his *Doctor From Lhasa* as remarkable, quoting and summarising from it across pages 44–45. Two pages on in *Breath of Life* (page 47), Day writes about Carl Reichenbach's debunked nineteenth-century theories of

Odic Force and as a true believer in pseudo-science opines: 'Others have called this force Ether, Bio-Cosmic Energy and Cosmic Orgone Energy; but call it what you will, it seems much the same thing as the *prana* of the Yogis.'

23. *Yoga For You* by Claude Bragdon, Andrew Dakers, London, not dated. The US edition published by Alfred A. Knopf, New York, is reported as dating from 1943.
24. *An Introduction To Yoga* by Claude Bragdon, Alfred A. Knopf, New York 1933.
25. Bragdon, *An Introduction To Yoga*, 7–8.
26. Bragdon, *Yoga For You*, v.
27. Bragdon, *Yoga For You*, 40–44, 44–48.
28. *Tantrik Yoga: Hindu & Tibetan* by J. Marques-Rivière, translated by H. E. Kennedy, Rider, London 1940.
29. 'Henri de Lubac et le xixe siècle comme symptôme' by Alain Rauwel, *Archives de sciences sociales des religions*, Vol. 172, No. 4, 2015, 193. Last accessed 25 November 2023: https://web.archive.org/web/20240819003022/https://journals.openedition.org/assr/27255
30. *The Inner Tradition And Yoga* by Charles Wase, Rider, London 1921, ix–x.
31. *Extra-Sensory Perception* by J. B. Rhine, Faber and Faber, London 1935. US edition Boston Society For Psychic Research, Boston, MA 1934. *Gland Treatment For Renewal Or Rejuvenation Of The Body Through Applied New Thought* by Grace Stuart, Elizabeth Towne Co., Holyoke, MA 1925.
32. *Yoga For The West* by Felix Guyot, translated by H. Bosman, Rider, London n.d. There was a US edition of this translation published by D. McKay of Philadelphia in 1934. Many sources give the UK publication date as 1937, but this seems to be an error.
33. Guyot, *Yoga For The West*, 105–106.
34. Guyot, *Yoga For The West*, 133.
35. Guyot, *Yoga For The West*, 125.
36. *Yogic Asanas for Health and Vigour* by V. G. Rele, D. B. Taraporevala Sons & Co., Bombay 1939. My page references are to the 1968 9th edition of the 1958 version of the book published by D. B. Taraporevala Sons & Co, Bombay. Rele's full name is Vasant Gangaram Rele. *The Mysterious Kundalini: The Physical Basis of the*

NOTES

'Kundali (Hatha) Yoga' in Terms of Western Anatomy and Physiology by Vasant G. Rele, D. B. Taraporevala Sons & Co., Bombay 1927, 2nd edition 1929, 3rd revised and enlarged edition 1931.
37. Rele, *Yogic Asanas for Health and Vigour*, 1–2.
38. *The Culture of the Abdomen: The Cure of Obesity and Constipation* by F. A. Hornibrook, William Heinemann, London 1924. My page references are to the 1957, Penguin, Harmondsworth, edition. This author's full name is Frederick Arthur Hornibrook. Found in the bibliographies of *Yogic Asanas for Health and Vigour*, 74 – this final page is unnumbered: Day, *The Study And Practice Of Yoga*, 158.
39. Hornibrook, *The Culture of the Abdomen*, 32–33.
40. Singleton, *Yoga Body*, 154–157.
41. His later yoga-related books included *Practical Yoga For Women* and *About Yoga Diet: The Eastern Way To Healthy Eating* by Harvey Day, Thorsons, Wellingborough, 1969.
42. Random examples: 'World Champion Had Psychic Sister-In-Law' by Harvey Day, *Prediction*, Vol. 26, No. 2, February 1960, 40–41; 'They Shall Not Die' by Harvey Day, *Prediction*, Vol. 28, No. 7, July 1962, 8, 9 and 24; 'Diagnosis By The Hand' by Harvey Day, *Prediction*, Vol. 28, No. 9, September 1962, 23–24; 'Ghost Country' by Harvey Day, *Prediction*, Vol. 32, No. 10, October 1966, 22–23.
43. *Yoga For Perfect Health* by 'Alain', Thorsons, London 1957. *Yoga The Amazing Life Science* by Major P. G. Francis, Thorsons, London 1958, who also authored *Streamlined Living: A Simple Yoga System For Success* by Major P. G. Francis (Late Indian Army), L. N. Fowler & Co, London not dated, and *Dynamic Yoga Is For You* by Philip G. Francis, A. Thomas, Preston, 1967.

11   Desmond Dunne aka Occultist James Lee-Richardson and His Mail Order Yoga Course

1. *The Manual And Who's Who Of Spiritualism And Psychic Research* edited and compiled by James Leigh, Francis Mott, London 1936. The Editor's Foreword to this compendium which concludes with the sign-off 'James Leigh, London, January 1st 1936', contains the following: 'Lastly, but by no means least emphasised, is my indebtedness to my colleague and fiancée, Miss M. Kemp … .' The England and Wales Civil Registration Marriage Index records

James Lee-Richardson and Minnie Kemp marrying in 1937. In the 1939 British census, they are recorded as living in the now abolished Municipal Borough of Malden and Coombe (which included New Malden) with their occupations being editor and housewife.

2. See *Insight School of Yoga Lessons* by Desmond Dunn, Insight School of Yoga, New Malden, not dated. The copy of the course held at the Paul Brunton Philosophic Foundation Archives carries the Insight House, New Malden, address associated with a number of Lee-Richardson business ventures.

3. On Jones' supplements, 'Labdoor's tests and reviews describe the products as little more than heavily overpriced supplements with few health benefits, if any. As Jones' popularity has risen, so has his supplements business, which sources have told BuzzFeed News largely funds Jones' highly controversial Infowars media empire ... .': 'We Sent Alex Jones' Infowars Supplements To A Lab. Here's What's In Them' by Charlie Warzel, *BuzzFeed News*, 9 August 2017. Last accessed 13 December 2024: http://web.archive.org/web/20241129225735/https://www.buzzfeednews.com/article/charliewarzel/we-sent-alex-jones-infowars-supplements-to-a-lab-heres

4. *Yoga for Everyman: How to Have Long Life and Happiness* by Desmond Dunne, Gerald Duckworth & Co, London 1951, front inside dust flap. On page 7, Lee-Richardson identifies his location as Insight House, New Malden.

5. See the cover of the American iteration of *Lesson 10* from his Insight School of Yoga mail order course: 'Concentration: Mind Control: Psychic Development'. On cost, see Newcombe, *Yoga in Britain*, 40–41: 'At this time (1956), he was charging £4 for the twelve-lesson course (equivalent to about £88 in 2018), requiring a correspondent with a certain amount of disposable income and ensuring some commitment to the course.'

6. Lee-Richardson, *Yoga For Everyman*, 110.

7. Lee-Richardson, *Yoga For Everyman*, 81–83.

8. Lee-Richardson, *Yoga For Everyman*, 101. The 'historic' poses are illustrated and described on pages 101–105.

9. Dunne, *Insight School of Yoga Lessons*, wrapper to *Lesson I*.

10. Dunne, *Insight School of Yoga Lessons*, *Lesson XII*, 4.

11. Dunne, *Insight School of Yoga Lessons*, *Lesson I*, 3.

Notes

12. Dunne, *Insight School of Yoga Lessons, Lesson XII*, 14.
13. Dunne, *Insight School of Yoga Lessons, Lesson I*, 12.
14. Dunne, *Insight School of Yoga Lessons, Lesson VII*, 4. Although found in medieval and early modern Christianity, the term 'Great Architect of the Universe' – abbreviated as both GAOTU and Great Architect – has in recent centuries been predominantly associated with Freemasonry. Given that within the English Masonic system, members must believe in a supreme creator, this term was used to refer to the deity without being denomination specific. Some claim the first appearance of the term in Masonic literature is found in the work James Anderson wrote for the English Grand Lodge under the title *The Constitutions of the Free-Masons* (1723). The term can be found on pages 7 and 25 of the 1734 edition published in Philadelphia by US founding father Benjamin Franklin (this was the first book on Freemasonry published in North America).
15. Dunne, *Insight School of Yoga Lessons, Lesson II*, 2–3.
16. Dunne, *Insight School of Yoga Lessons, Lesson II*, 6.
17. Dunne, *Insight School of Yoga Lessons, Lesson III*, 7.
18. A 2021 *Wired* article points to Guru Jagat, Bizzie Gold, Stephanie Birch, Sayer Ji, Kelly Brogan and Krystal Tini as yoga influencers who have promoted anti-vax and related conspiracy theories. See 'The Yoga World Is Riddled With Anti-Vaxxers and QAnon Believers' by Cécile Guerin, *Wired*, 28 January 2021.
19. Dunne, *Insight School of Yoga Lessons, Lesson III*, 2–3.
20. Dunne, *Insight School of Yoga Lessons, Lesson IV*, 5 and 8.
21. Dunne, *Insight School of Yoga Lessons, Lesson VI*, 6–9.
22. Newcombe, *Yoga in Britain*, 220.
23. Newcombe, *Yoga in Britain*, 39.
24. Newcombe, *Yoga in Britain*, 248, states in her footnotes: 'A Mass Observation archivist was unable to find any record of this research in the MO Archive at the University of Sussex noting that they only have incomplete records dating after 1949 when the organization began taking private commissions.'
25. Lee-Richardson, *Yoga For Everyman*, 22–23.
26. *Fate Magazine* (UK edition), Vol. 1, No. 3, January 1955, Worcester Park, Surrey, 81.
27. *The Manual Of Yoga* by Desmond Dunne, W. Foulsham & Co, London 1956. Lee-Richardson also did a follow-up book to *The*

Manual Of Yoga for the same publisher entitled *The Manual Of Hypnotism* by Desmond Dunne, W. Foulsham & Co, London 1959.
28. Dunne, *Manual Of Yoga*, 72.
29. Dunne, *Yoga Made Easy*, 142.
30. See, for example, credits on contents page (unnumbered) of *Fate*, Vol. 1 No. 2, December 1954, Press Books Ltd, Worcester Park, Surrey. The editor is given as James Leigh and associate editors include Adrienne Arden. Lee-Richardson uses his legal name as editor-in-chief for *Here's Health* – see, for example, *Here's Health Family Guide For 1959*, Press Books Ltd, Worcester Park, Surrey.
31. See 'Insight Institute Tarot Course' by Auntie Tarot, *Auntie's Tarot Blog*, 13 July 2011; 'Insight Institute Tarot Course – Update' by Auntie Tarot, *Auntie's Tarot Blog*, 17 July 2011, and *The Insight Institute* by Auntie Tarot, *Auntie's Tarot Blog*, 11 September 2011 – links below. The first post dates an ad for the Insight Institute in *Prediction*, December 1947. The third post reproduces the ad and reveals that at the end of 1947 the address of the Insight Institute was 20 Blackfriars Lane, London EC4. The second post dates a second *Prediction* ad for the Insight Institute to October 1948. The third post reproduces this ad and shows that at the time the Insight Institute address was Insight House, New Malden, Surrey. The third post also reproduces an ad from the 1954 *Prediction Annual*, which may date from the end of 1953, which gives the address of the Insight Institute as Manor House, Worcester Park, Surrey. Last accessed 1 December 2023, achieved here: https://web.archive.org/web/20231201212236/https://auntietarot.wordpress.com/2011/07/13/insight-institute-tarot-course/

Here: https://web.archive.org/web/20231201213337/https://auntietarot.wordpress.com/2011/07/17/insight-institute-tarot-course-update/

And here: https://web.archive.org/web/20231201210807/https://auntietarot.wordpress.com/2011/09/11/the-insight-institute/
32. 'Insight Institute' by Simon Wintle, *World Of Playing Cards* website, 11 January 2013. Last accessed 13 November 2023: https://web.archive.org/web/20230321053934/https://www.wopc.co.uk/tarot/insight-institute

33. Her signature is visible on a photograph showing a welcome letter to the tarot course – although the auctioneer who put this online has mistranscribed her surname. Last accessed 1 December 2023: https://web.archive.org/web/20231121114248/https://www.easyliveauction.com/catalogue/lot/3d4692288bf1d21 6d22a06eea6f02572/0af8d24542e81eb9357e7ef448a6646f/general-sales-including-collectables-furniture-and-jew-lot-129/
34. See, for example, *Prediction*, Vol. 1, No. 1, London, February 1936, page 1 which lists James Leigh as editor and features an article entitled 'How To Read Your Hand' by Noel Jacquin on pages 20–30.
35. *My Occult Case Book* by Frank Lind, Rider, London 1953, ix.
36. *Palmistry For Everyone: An Outline of Chirology* by Vera Compton, Duckworth, London 1952.
37. See '5 Fake Photos That Once Fooled Everyone But Now Fool Only Fools' by Katie Serena, *All That's Interesting*, 20 October 2017. Last accessed 1 December 2023: https://web.archive.org/web/20230201191640/https://allthatsinteresting.com/famous-fake-photos/3
38. An Insight Institute ad in the UK *Fate*, Vol. 1, No. 3, January 1955, Press Books, Worcester Park, Surrey, 96, offers the following courses for £2 each: 'How To Cast Horoscopes', 'How To Read Horoscopes', 'How To Analyse Handwriting', 'How To Read Tarot', 'How To Read Hands', 'Advanced Hand Reading', 'How To Develop Psychic Powers'.
39. *Prediction*, edited by James Leigh, Vol. 1, 1936, published from Link House, 4–8 Greville Street, London EC1.
40. 'I Interview An Indian Yogi! My Meeting With The Most Famous Occultist In All India' by Paul Brunton, *Prediction*, Vol. 1, No. 6, July 1936, 258–260.
41. 'Strange Feats Of The Yogis' by Pundit Dinkarswami, *Prediction*, Vol. 1, No. 6, July 1936, 283–284; *Prediction*, Vol. 1, No. 6, July 1936, 271–272.
42. *Here's Health Family Health Guide for 1959*, Press Books, Manor House, Worcester Park, Surrey, 1959. The credits on page 7 include J. Lee-Richardson editor-in-chief, E Gilbert Oakley editor, and J. Lee-Richardson publisher.

12 Richard Hittleman and Yogic Televangelism

1. Linda Hittleman quoted in the feature 'Death and Taxes: When famed American yoga guru Richard Hittleman died in Santa Cruz in 1991, he left his ex-wife with a million-dollar tax bill, merciless IRS agents at the door and nowhere to turn' by Ami Chen Mills, *Metro*, 22–29 November 1995. Last accessed 2 December 2023, archived here: https://web.archive.org/web/20000123082059/http://www.metroactive.com/papers/metro/11.22.95/yogi-9547.html
2. *Guide To Yoga Meditation* by Richard Hittleman, Bantam Books, New York 1969, 10–14.
3. *Guide For The Seeker* by Richard Hittleman, Bantam Books, New York 1978, 92.
4. *Yoga For Health* by Richard Hittleman, Hamlyn, London 1989 edition (originally published 1971).
5. Mills, 'Death and Taxes'.
6. Newcombe, *Yoga in Britain*, 151.
7. *Be Young With Yoga* by Richard Hittleman, Prentice Hall, Englewood Cliffs, NJ 1962, sixth printing February 1971; *Yoga For Physical Fitness* by Richard Hittleman, Prentice Hall, Englewood Cliff, NJ, 1964, third printing September 1966.
8. Hittleman, *Guide For The Seeker*, 159.
9. Hittleman, *Guide To Yoga Meditation*, 12–13.
10. Hittleman, *Be Young With Yoga*, 221.
11. Hittleman, *Yoga For Physical Fitness*, 150–151; *Functional Anatomy of the Spine* by Alison Middleditch and Jean Oliver, Elsevier, London 2005, 2nd edition, 153–172.
12. *Yoga Philosophy & Meditation: An Interpretation* by Richard L. Hittleman, privately published, Hollywood, CA 1964, 19.
13. Hittleman, *Guide To Yoga Meditation*, 103.
14. *Yoga: The 8 Steps To Health And Peace* by Richard Hittleman, Bantam Press, New York 1976, 77. Original Deerfield Communications Corporation edition published 1975.
15. Hittleman, *Yoga: The 8 Steps To Health And Peace*, 36.
16. Bragdon, *Yoga For You*, 12.
17. Hittleman, *Yoga Philosophy & Meditation*, 13. The story is repeated in Hittleman, *Guide To Yoga Meditation*, 66–67.

18. Mills, 'Death and Taxes'.
19. Mills, 'Death and Taxes'.
20. Mills, 'Death and Taxes'.
21. 'Preaching Fascism: Inside San Diego's Awaken Megachurch' by Kate Burns, *Left Coast Right Watch*, 21 February 2023. Last accessed 14 December 2024: http://web.archive.org/web/20240618173214/https://leftcoastrightwatch.org/articles/preaching-fascism-inside-san-diegos-awaken-megachurch/

13 Pull the Wool Over Your Own Eyes with Frank Rudolph Young, the 'Einstein' of Occult Yoga

1. *Psychic City Chicago: Doorway To Another Dimension* by Brad Steiger, Doubleday, New York 1976, 124.
2. A six-hour audio-book version of Frank Rudolph Young's *Cyclomancy* uploaded to YouTube by Stargate Books in 2023 has had over 100,000 hits in just over a year. Last accessed 14 December 2024: http://web.archive.org/web/20241214232754/https://www.youtube.com/watch?v=PxpiifkgL8Q
3. Steiger, *Psychic City Chicago*, 133.
4. *The Yogatronic Diet: Amazing New Way To A Youthful, Trim Body* by Frank Rudolph Young, Parker Publishing, West Nyack, NY 1979, 43.
5. 'Dr. Frank Rudolph Young and Yogametrics' by Greg Joel Newton, not dated. Last accessed 13 June 2023, archived here: https://web.archive.org/web/20160906043702/http://www.focusedmusculartension.com/dr-frank-rudolph-young
6. *Cyclomancy – The Secret of Psychic Power Control* by Frank Rudolph Young, Parker Publishing Company, West Nyack, NY 1966, iii.
7. *Yoga Secrets For Extraordinary Health & Long Life* by Frank Rudolph Young, Parker Publishing, West Nyack, NY 1976, 217; *Solar Diet. The Secrets of Wise Eating* by Rex Grant, Solar Health, Chicago, IL 1955.
8. Last accessed 14 July 2023, archived here: https://web.archive.org/web/20220719114208/http://www.copyrightencyclopedia.com/cobra-self-defense-street-fighting-tricks-designed-to-help/ – and also, last accessed 14 July 2023, archived here: https://web.archive.org/web/20230614211355/https://books.google.

co.uk/books/about/Solar_Diet_The_Secrets_of_Wise_Eating. html?id=1ev7MgEACAAJ&redir_esc=y

9. *X-Ray Mind: A Krishnara Course* by Maravedi El Krishnar, Krishnar Institute of Universal Knowledge, Escondido, CA 1953. Young's copyright registrations include the pseudonym Maravedi El Krishnar. *Catalog of Copyright Entries. Third Series: 1953: January–June* by Library of Congress Copyright Office (1954, p. 590), lists Young as the author of *X-Ray Mind* under the pseudonym Maravedi El Krishnar.
10. Krishnar, *X-Ray Mind*, 7–8.
11. Krishnar, *X-Ray Mind*, 109.
12. Krishnar, *X-Ray Mind*, 121.
13. Krishnar, *X-Ray Mind*, 123.
14. *How To Pick Up Girls* by Eric Weber, Symphony Press, Tenafly, NJ 1970; *The Art of Erotic Seduction* by Albert Ellis and Roger Conway, L. Stuart, New York 1967.
15. Krishnar, *X-Ray Mind*, 130–131.
16. *The Laws Of Mental Domination: How to master and use them for dynamic life force* by Frank Rudolph Young, Parker Publishing, West Nyack, NY 1965.
17. Young, *Laws of Mental Domination*, viii.
18. Young, *Cyclomancy*, 14.
19. *The Secrets Of Personal Psychic Power* by Frank Rudolph Young, Parker Publishing, West Nyack, NY 1967.
20. See commentary on Indra Devi's Prentice Hall books above. Two further random examples: *The Magic Power Of Pragma-Psychics* by Tom C. Lyle, Parker Publishing Company, West Nyack, NY 1970, and *Doctor Cantor's Secrets Of Self-Revitalization* by Alfred J. Cantor, MD, Parker Publishing Company, West Nyack, NY 1979.
21. *The Secrets Of Personal Psychic Power* by Frank Rudolph Young, Parker Publishing, West Nyack, NY 1967, 12.
22. *Psychastra: Key To Secret ESP + Control* by Frank Rudolph Young, Parker Publishing, West Nyack, NY 1968, dust jacket front inner sleeve.
23. *Yoga For Men Only* by Frank Rudolph Young, Parker Publishing, West Nyack, NY 1969, v and 1.
24. Young, *Yoga For Men Only*, 134.
25. Young, *Yoga For Men Only*, 136.

26. Young, *Yoga For Men Only*, 158. Similar advice to Young's on backbends can be found in reputable sources such as *Surviving Exercise: Judy Alter's Safe and Sane Exercise Program* by Judy Alter, Houghton Mifflin Company, Boston, MA 1983.
27. Young, *Yoga For Men Only*, 87–89.
28. Young, *Yoga Secrets For Extraordinary Health*, 193.
29. Young, *Yoga Secrets For Extraordinary Health*, 180.
30. Young, *Cyclomancy*, 130.
31. *Zodiac Force Control: Secret of Miracle Healing and Long Life* by Frank Rudolph Young, Parker Publishing, West Nyack, NY 1977, 9.
32. Young, *Zodiac Force Control*, 22–23.
33. Young, *Zodiac Force Control*, 117–122.
34. Young, *Zodiac Force Control*, 116.
35. *The Yogatronic Diet: Amazing New Way to a Youthful, Trim Body* by Frank Rudolph Young, Parker Publishing Company, West Nyack, NY 1979.
36. Young, *Yogatronic Diet*, 42.
37. Young, *Yogatronic Diet*, 42.
38. *Fads And Fallacies In The Name Of Science* by Martin Gardner, Dover Publications, New York 1957, footnote p. 345.
39. Young, *Yogatronic Diet*, 50.
40. See, for example, the video *Cyclomancy Day 1* by Occult Nachos, 'posted 1 year ago', last accessed 27 June 2023, archived here: https://web.archive.org/web/20230627224329/https://www.youtube.com/watch?v=UjbmoCcgoeU
41. See *Clown World: Four Years Inside Andrew Tate's Manosphere* by Jamie Tahsin and Matt Shea, Quercus, London 2024.

Conclusion

1. 'New investigation for BBC Sounds and Radio 4 uncovers shocking allegations of sexual exploitation, grooming and trafficking linked to a yoga movement with followers in the UK, as British woman speaks out against accused guru Gregorian Bivolaru' by Anon., *BBC* website, 9 December 2024. Last accessed 15 December 2024: http://web.archive.org/web/20241210113218/https://www.bbc.co.uk/mediacentre/2024/world-of-secrets-the-bad-guru

2. '"There's no going back": A survivor's story of a cult's manipulation and exploitation' by Charlie Lewis, *Crikey*, 27 September 2024. Last accessed 15 December 2024: http://web.archive.org/web/20241212192933/https://www.crikey.com.au/2024/09/27/cult-misa-survivor-story/
3. 'Tantric Yoga Guru Gregorian Bivolaru Charged With Human Trafficking', *The Guardian*, 28 November 2023. Last accessed 15 December 2024: http://web.archive.org/web/20241129235331/https://www.theguardian.com/world/2023/nov/28/tantric-yoga-guru-gregorian-bivolaru-charged-with-human-trafficking
4. 'Fears Mount Over Scale Of Buddhist Sect Sexual Abuse. Followers allege they were coerced into sex in 1970s and 80s with elders of UK's Triratna order' by Jamie Doward, *The Guardian*, 19 February 2017. Last accessed 26 October 2024: http://web.archive.org/web/20170219024542/https://www.theguardian.com/world/2017/feb/19/buddhist-sexual-abuse-triratna-dennis-lingwood
5. A fraudulent 1998 medical study authored by Andrew Wakefield and others linked the MMR (measles, mumps and rubella) vaccine to autism in children and led to a significant decline in vaccination. The paper was subsequently discredited by a series of studies but even after it was withdrawn, anti-vax fanatics continued repeating its false claims. Journalist Brian Deer subsequently exposed those behind the study as having falsified its results, their motive being financial gain. See 'Wakefield's Article Linking MMR Vaccine and Autism was Fraudulent', editorial by Fiona Godlee and colleagues, *British Medical Journal*, 6 January 2011. Last accessed 14 January 2025: http://web.archive.org/web/20250101132337/https://www.bmj.com/content/342/bmj.c7452
6. 'A Sydney Yoga Studio Compared Fully Vaxxed Freedoms To Segregation' by Millie Roberts, *Junkee*, 7 October 2021. Last accessed 10 December 2024: http://web.archive.org/web/20211007031727/https://junkee.com/yoga-vaccination-sydney/310905
7. 'The High-Profile Sydney Yoga Studio At The Centre Of A Decidedly Un-Zen Scandal' by Sally Rawsthorne, *Sydney Morning Herald*, 26 May 2024. Last accessed 10 December 2024: http://web.archive.org/web/20240526063303/https://www.smh.com.

au/national/nsw/the-high-profile-sydney-yoga-studio-at-the-centre-of-a-decidedly-un-zen-scandal-20240526-p5jgpm.html

Bibliography

Books and Pamphlets

Alain: *Yoga For Perfect Health*, Thorsons, London 1957.

Alter, Judy: *Surviving Exercise: Judy Alter's Safe and Sane Exercise Program*, Houghton Mifflin Company, Boston, MA 1983.

Anderson, James: T*he Constitutions of the Free-Masons*, privately published, Philadelphia, PA 1734.

Anon., ed.: *The Spectator Booklets 1: Parliament Or Dictatorship?* Methuen & Company, London 1934.

Arden, Adrienne: *How To Know Your Future*, Bazaar, Exchange & Mart, London 1951.

Bartolini, Simonetta: *Yoga. Sovversivi e rivoluzionari con d'Annunzio a Fiume*, Luni Editrice, Milan 2019.

Behanan, Kovoor T: *Yoga: A Scientific Evaluation*, Secker & Warburg, London 1938.

Beres, Derek, Remski, Matthew and Walker, Julian: *Conspirituality: How New Age Conspiracy Theories Became A Health Threat*, Public Affairs, New York 2023.

Berghaus, Günter: *Futurism and Politics: Between Anarchist Rebellion and Fascist Reaction, 1909–1944*, Berghahn Books, Oxford 1995.

Bernard, Theos: *Hatha Yoga: The Report of a Personal Experience*, Rider & Company, London 1950.

Bradgon, Claude: *An Introduction To Yoga*, Alfred A. Knopf, New York 1933.

Bragdon, Claude: *Yoga For You*, Andrew Dakers, London, not dated, circa 1943.

Brunton, Paul: *The Quest Of The Overself*, Rider, London 1937.

Buckland, Raymond: *The Magic Of Chantomatics*, Parker Publishing, West Nyack, NY 1978.

Cantor, Alfred J., MD: *Doctor Cantor's Secrets Of Self-Revitalization*, Parker Publishing Company, West Nyack, NY 1979.

BIBLIOGRAPHY

Compton, Vera: *Palmistry For Everyone: An Outline of Chirology*, Duckworth, London 1952.

Day, Harvey: *About Yoga: The Complete Philosophy*, Thorsons, London 1951.

Day, Harvey: *The Study and Practice Of Yoga*, Thorsons, London 1953.

Day, Harvey: *You, Too, Can Write For Money*, A. Thomas, Preston 1961.

Day, Harvey: *The Breath Of Life*, Thorsons, London 1965.

Day, Harvey: *Seeing Into The Future*, Thorsons, London 1966.

Day, Harvey: *Handbook Of Hypnosis*, Thorsons, London 1967.

Day, Harvey: *Practical Yoga*, Thorsons, London 1967.

Day, Harvey: *About Yoga Diet: The Eastern Way To Healthy Eating*, Thorsons, Wellingborough, 1969.

Day, Harvey: *Practical Yoga For Women*, Pelham Books, London 1969.

Day, Harvey: *Luck Of The Toss*, Pelham Books, London, 1970.

Day, Harvey: *Practical Yoga For The Businessman*, Pelham Books, London 1970.

Day, Harvey: *Yoga Illustrated Dictionary*, Kaye and Ward, London 1971.

Day, Harvey: *Karma Yoga: The Philosophy of Contentment*, Aquarian Press, Wellingborough 1972.

Day, Harvey: *Yoga For The Athlete*, Kaye and Ward, London 1974.

Day, Harvey: *Occult Illustrated Dictionary*, Kaye & Ward Ltd, London 1975.

Day, Harvey: *Encyclopaedia Of Natural Health and Healing*, Kaye & Ward Ltd, London 1979.

Day, Harvey: *Into The Unknown*, Bishopsgate Press, London 1987.

Delaney, Walter (Pseud Joseph Schaumberger): *Ultra-Psychonics: How to Work Miracles with the Limitless Power of Psycho-Atomic Energy*, Parker Publishing, West Nyack, NY 1975.

De Michelis, Elizabeth: *A History of Modern Yoga: Patanjali and Western Esotericism*, Continuum, London & New York 2004.

Devi, Indra: *Forever Young, Forever Healthy*, A. Thomas & Co, London 1955.

Devi, Indra: *Yoga For Americans: A Complete 6 Weeks' Course for Home Practice*, Prentice Hall, Englewood Cliffs, NJ 1959.

Devi, Indra: *Renew Your Life Through Yoga*, Paperback Library, New York 1969.

Devi, Savitri: *The Lightning and the Sun*, self-published by the author, Calcutta 1958.

Djurdjevic, Gordan: *India and the Occult: The Influence of South Asian Spirituality on Modern Western Occultism*, Palgrave Macmillan, London 2014.

Dukes, Paul: *The Unending Quest: Autobiographical Sketches*, Cassell & Co., London 1950.

Dukes, Paul: *Yoga For The Western World*, privately published by Students of Western Yoga, place of publication not listed, 1959.

Dukes, Paul: *The Yoga of Health, Youth and Joy: A Treatise On Hatha Yoga Adapted To The West*, Cassell, London 1960.

Duncan, Derek: *Reading and Writing Italian Homosexuality: A Case of Possible Difference*, Ashgate, Aldershot 2006.

Dunne, Desmond (Pseud James Lee-Richardson): *Yoga for Everyman: How to Have Long Life and Happiness*, Gerald Duckworth & Co. Ltd, London 1951.

Dunne, Desmond (Pseud James Lee-Richardson): *The Manual Of Yoga*, W. Foulsham & Co, London 1956.

Dunne, Desmond (Pseud James Lee-Richardson): *The Manual Of Hypnotism*, W. Foulsham & Co, London 1959.

Dunne, Desmond (Pseud James Lee-Richardson): *Yoga Made Easy*, Prentice Hall, Englewood Cliffs, NJ 1961.

Ehrenreich, Barbara: *Smile Or Die: How Positive Thinking Fooled America & The World*, Granta Books, London 2009.

Eliade, Mircea: *Yoga: Immortality and Freedom*, translated by Willard R. Trask, Princeton University Press, Princeton, NJ 1970, paperback edition.

Ellis, Albert and Conway, Roger: *The Art of Erotic Seduction*, L. Stuart, New York 1967.

Evola, Julius: *The Yoga of Power: Tantra, Shakti, and the Secret Way*, Inner Traditions, Rochester 1992.

Feuerstein, Georg: *The Essence of Yoga: A contribution to the Psychohistory of Indian Civilisation*, Rider, London 1974.

Feuerstein, Georg: *The Yoga Tradition: Its History, Literature, Philosophy and Practice*, Hohm Press, Prescott, AZ, new edition 2001.

Feuerstein, Georg and Payne, Larry: *Yoga For Dummies*, Wiley Publishing, Hoboken, NJ 1999.

BIBLIOGRAPHY

Francis, P. G.: *Streamlined Living : A Simple Yoga System For Success*, L. N. Fowler & Co, London, not dated circa 1940s.

Francis, P. G.: *Yoga The Amazing Life Science*, Thorsons, London 1958.

Francis, P. G.: *Dynamic Yoga Is For You*, A. Thomas, Preston 1967.

Friend, John: *Anusara Yoga Teacher Training Manual*, Anusara Press, Texas 2005, updated seventh edition.

Fuller, J. F. C.: *The Star in the West: A Critical Essay Upon the Works of Aleister Crowley*, Walter Scott Publishing Company, London 1907.

Fuller, J. F. C.: *Yoga: A Study of the Mystical Philosophy of the Brahmins and Buddhists*, Rider, London 1925.

Gardner, Martin: *Fads And Fallacies In The Name Of Science*, Dover Publications, New York 1957.

Goldberg, Elliott: *The Path of Modern Yoga: The History of an Embodied Spiritual Practice*, Inner Traditions, Rochester, VT 2016.

Goldberg, Michelle: *The Goddess Pose: The Audacious Life of Indra Devi, The Woman Who Helped Bring Yoga To The West*, Corsair, London 2016.

Goodrick-Clarke, Nicholas: *The Occult Roots of Nazism: The Ariosophists of Austria and Germany, 1890–1935*, New York University Press, New York 1993.

Goodrich-Clarke, Nicholas: *Hitler's Priestess: Savitri Devi, the Hindu-Aryan Myth, and Neo-Nazism*, New York University Press, New York 2000.

Goodrich-Clarke, Nicholas: *Black Sun: Aryan Cults, Esoteric Nazism, and the Politics of Identity*, New York University Press, New York 2002.

Gray-Cobb, Geof: *Secrets From Beyond the Pyramids: How to Gain Control of Your Destiny*, Parker Publishing, West Nyack NY 1979.

Guyot, Felix: *Yoga For The West*, translated by H. Bosman, Rider, London not dated circa 1934.

Guyot, Felix: *Yoga: The Science of Health*, translated by J. Carling, Rider, London 1937.

Hackett, Paul G.: *Theos Bernard, The White Lama: Tibet, Yoga, and American Religious Life*, Columbia University Press, New York 2012.

Hettinger, Theodor and Thurlwell, M. H.: *Physiology of Strength*, Charles C. Thomas, Springfield, IL 1961.

Hittleman, Richard: *Be Young With Yoga*, Prentice Hall, Englewood Cliffs, NJ 1962.

Hittleman, Richard: *Yoga For Physical Fitness*, Prentice Hall, Englewood Cliffs, NJ, 1964.

Hittleman, Richard: *Yoga Philosophy & Meditation: An Interpretation*, privately published, Hollywood, CA 1964.

Hittleman, Richard: *Yoga USA*, Bantam Books, New York 1968.

Hittleman, Richard: *Guide To Yoga Mediation*, Bantam Books, New York 1969.

Hittleman, Richard: *Yoga: The 8 Steps To Health And Peace*, Bantam Books, New York 1976.

Hittleman, Richard: *Guide For The Seeker*, Bantam Books, New York 1978.

Hittleman, Richard: *Yoga For Health*, Hamlyn, London 1989.

Hornibrook, F. A.: *The Culture of the Abdomen: The Cure of Obesity and Constipation*, William Heinemann, London 1924.

Hornibrook, F. A.: *Live Without Tension*, Souvenir Press, London 1958.

Hutton, Ronald: *The Triumph of the Moon: A History of Modern Pagan Witchcraft*, Oxford University Press, 1999.

Jackson, Mark and Moore, Martin D., eds: *Balancing The Self: Medicine, Politics and the Regulation of Health in the Twentieth Century*, Manchester University Press 2020.

Jansa, Janez and Quaranta, Domenico: *Seaport Of Love*, translated by Anna Carruthers, Aksioma – Institute for Contemporary Art, Ljubljana 2009.

Jha, Dwijendra Narayan: *The Myth of the Holy Cow*, Verso, London 2002.

Kaye, Jacqueline, ed.: *Ezra Pound And America*, Palgrave Macmillan, London 1992.

Krishnar, Maravedi El (Pseud Frank Rudolph Young): *X-Ray Mind: A Krishnara Course*, Institute of Universal Knowledge, Escondido, CA 1953.

Krishnar, Maravedi El (Pseud Frank Rudolph Young): *Miracle Mind: Acquire The Mind Of A Genius, Course 1–2*, Institute of Universal Knowledge, no place of publication indicated 1954.

Ledeen, Michael A.: *The First Duce: d'Annunzio at Fiume*, Transaction Publishers, New Brunswick, NJ, 3rd edition 2009.

Lee-Richardson, J.: *Outboard Boating*, Arco Publications, London 1962.

BIBLIOGRAPHY

Lee-Richardson, J. and Oakley, Gilbert E., eds: *Here's Health Family Health Guide for 1959*, Press Books, Worcester Park, Surrey 1959.

Leigh, James (Pseud James Lee-Richardson), ed./compiler: *The Manual And Who's Who Of Spiritualism And Psychic Research*, Francis Mott, London 1936.

Leigh, James (Pseud James Lee-Richardson): *How To Apply Numerology*, Bazaar, Exchange & Mart, London 1951.

Lind, Frank: *How To Understand The Tarot*, Bazaar, Exchange and Mart, London 1952.

Lind, Frank: *My Occult Case Book*, Rider, London 1953.

Love, Robert: *The Great Oom: The Improbable Birth of Yoga in America*, Viking, New York 2010.

Lyle, Tom C.: *The Magic Power Of Pragma-Psychics*, Parker Publishing Company, West Nyack, NY 1970.

Marquès-Rivière, J.: *Tantrik Yoga: Hindu & Tibetan*, translated by H. E. Kennedy, Rider, London 1940.

Marsh, Alec: *John Kasper and Ezra Pound: Saving the Republic*, Bloomsbury, London 2015.

McLaurin, Hamish: *Eastern Philosophy For Western Minds*, The Stratford Company, Boston, MA 1933.

Middleditch, Alison and Oliver, Jean: *Functional Anatomy of the Spine*, Elsevier, London 2005, 2nd edition.

Montalban, Madeline: *Prediction Book Of The Tarot*, Blandford, London 1983.

Newcombe, Suzanne: *Yoga in Britain: Stretching Spirituality and Educating Yogis*, Equinox, Sheffield, 2019.

Norris, P. E. (Pseud Harvey Day): *About Honey: Nature's Elixir for Health and Energy*, Thorsons, London 1954.

Norris, P. E. (Pseud Harvey Day): *About Yeast, A Unique and Concentrated Natural Food*, Thorsons, London 1954.

Norris, P. E. (Pseud Harvey Day): *About Yogurt: An Invaluable Aid To Health*, Thorsons, London 1954.

Paramahamsa, Mahatma Agamya: *Sri Brahma Dhara: Shower From The Highest Through The Favour Of The Mahatma Sri Agamya Guru Paramahamsa*, Luzac & Company, London 1905.

Patanjali, Bhagwan Shree: *Aphorisms of Yoga*, translated by Shree Purohit Swami, Faber & Faber, London 1938.

Poewe, Karla: *New Religions and the Nazis*, Routledge, Oxon 2006.

Purohit, Swami Shree, translator: *The Ten Principal Upanishads*, Faber & Faber, London 1937.

Ramacharaka, Yogi (Pseud William Walker Atkinson): *Fourteen Lessons In Yogic Philosophy and Oriental Occultism*, Yogic Publication Society, Chicago. IL 1903.

Ramacharaka, Yogi (Pseud William Walker Atkinson): *The Hindu-Yogi Science Of Breath: A Complete Manual of the Oriental Breathing Philosophy of Physical, Mental, Psychic and Spiritual Development*, Yogic Publication Society, Chicago, IL 1903.

Ramacharaka, Yogi (Pseud William Walker Atkinson): *Hatha Yoga*, Yogi Publishing Society, Chicago, IL 1904.

Rampa, T. Lobsang (Pseud. Cyril Henry Hoskin): *Doctor from Lhasa*, Souvenir Press, London 1959.

Rele, V. G.: *Yogic Asanas for Health and Vigour*, D. B. Taraporevala Sons & Co., Bombay 1939.

Rele, V. G.: *The Mysterious Kundalini: The Physical Basis of the 'Kundali (Hatha) Yoga' in Terms of Western Anatomy and Physiology*, D. B. Taraporevala Sons & Co., Bombay 1927.

Remski, Matthew: *Practice And All Is Coming: Abuse, Cult Dynamics And Healing In Yoga And Beyond*, Embodied Wisdom Publishing, Rangiora 2019.

Rhine, J.B.: *Extra-Sensory Perception*, Faber and Faber, London 1935.

Sedgwick, Mark: *Against the Modern World: Traditionalism and the Secret Intellectual History of the Twentieth Century*, Oxford University Press, 2004.

Singleton, Mark: *Yoga Body: The Origins of Modern Posture Practice*, Oxford University Press, 2010.

Serrano, Miguel: *Adolf Hitler, el Último Avatāra*, La Nueva Edad, Santiago 1984.

Sivananda, Swarmi: *Yogic Home Exercises. Easy Course of Physical Culture for Men & Women*, Taraporevala Sons & Co., Bombay 1944.

Stanfield, Paul Scott: *Yeats and Politics in the 1930s*, Palgrave Macmillan, London 1988.

Steiger, Brad: *Psychic City Chicago: Doorway To Another Dimension*, Doubleday, New York 1976.

Sternhell, Zeev: *The Birth of Fascist Ideology*, Princeton University Press, Princeton, NJ 1989.

Stuart, Grace: *Gland Treatment For Renewal Or Rejuvenation Of The Body Through Applied New Thought*, Elizabeth Towne Co, Holyoke, MA 1925.

Sundaram, Yogacharya: *The Secret of Happiness Or Yogic Physical Culture*, 8th edition revised, Yoga Publishing House, Coimbatore 2000.

Syman, Stefanie: *The Subtle Body: The Story of Yoga In America*, Farrar, Straus & Giroux, New York 2010.

Sunshine, Spencer: *Neo-Nazi Terrorism and Countercultural Fascism: The Origins and Afterlife of James Mason's Siege*, Routledge, Oxfordshire 2024.

Tahsin, Jamie and Shea, Matt: *Clown World: Four Years Inside Andrew Tate's Manosphere*, Quercus, London 2024.

Thorsson, Edred (Pseud Stephen Flowers): *Rune Might: The Secret Practices of the German Rune Magicians*, Inner Traditions, Rochester, VT 2019.

Tietke, Mathias: *Yoga im Nationalsozialismus: Konzepte, Kontraste, Konsequenzen*, Ludwig, Kiel 2011.

Treviso, Luigi Urettin: *Giovanni Comisso, Un provinciale in fuga*, Istresco, 2009.

Tryphonopoulos, Demetres P.: *The Celestial Tradition: A Study of Ezra Pound's The Cantos*, Wilfrid Laurier University Press, Ontario 1992.

Veenhof, Douglas: *White Lama: The Life of Tantric Yogi Theos Bernard, Tibet's Emissary to the New World*, Harmony Books, New York 2011.

Wase, Charles: *The Inner Tradition And Yoga*, Rider, London 1921.

Weber, Eric: *How To Pick Up Girls*, Symphony Press, Tenafly, NJ 1970.

White, David Gordon, ed.: *Yoga In Practice*, Princeton University Press, Princeton, NJ 2012.

White, David Gordon: *The Yoga Sutra of Patanjali: A Biography*, Princeton University Press, Princeton, NJ 2014.

Woodhouse, John: *Gabriele D'Annunzio: Defiant Archangel*, Oxford University Press, 2001.

Wrench, Evelyn: *Francis Yeats-Brown 1886–1944*, Eyre and Spottiswoode, London 1948.

Yeats-Brown, Francis: *Caught By The Turks*, Arnold, London 1919.

Yeats-Brown, Francis: *Star and Crescent: Being the Story of the 17th Cavalry from 1858 to 1922*, Naval and Military Press 2009. Privately published 1927.

Yeats-Brown, Francis: *Bengal Lancer*, Gollancz, London 1930.

Yeats-Brown, Francis: *Golden Horn*, Gollancz, London 1932.

Yeats-Brown, Francis: *The Eight Steps To Yoga As Told To Otis Peabody Swift*, Blue Ribbon Books, New York 1933.

Yeats-Brown, Francis, ed.: *Escape. A Book of Escapes of All Kinds*, Eyre & Spottiswoode, London 1933.

Yeats-Brown, Francis: *Dogs of War*, Peter Davis, London 1934.

Yeats-Brown, Francis: *Lancer At Large*, Gollancz, London 1936.

Yeats-Brown, Francis: *Yoga Explained*, Gollancz, London 1937.

Yeats-Brown, Francis: *European Jungle*, Eyre & Spottiswoode, London 1939.

Yesudian, Selvarajan and Haich, Elisabeth: *Yoga And Health*, George Allen & Unwin, London 1953.

Young, Frank Rudolph: *Dr. Young's Stop Stammering Part 1, Part 2 & Part 3*, Gaucho, Chicago, IL 1962.

Young, Frank Rudolph: *The Laws Of Mental Domination: How to master and use them for dynamic life force*, Parker Publishing, West Nyack, NY 1965.

Young, Frank Rudolph: *Cyclomancy – The Secret of Psychic Power Control*, Parker Publishing Company, West Nyack, NY 1966.

Young, Frank Rudolph: *The Secrets Of Personal Psychic Power*, Parker Publishing, West Nyack, NY 1967.

Young, Frank Rudolph: *Psychastra: Key To Secret ESP + Control*, Parker Publishing, West Nyack, NY 1968.

Young, Frank Rudolph: *Yoga For Men Only*, Parker Publishing, West Nyack, NY 1969.

Young, Frank Rudolph: *The Secret Of Spirit Thought Magic*, Parker Publishing, West Nyack, NY 1971.

Young, Frank Rudolph: *Secret Mental Powers: Miracle of Mind Magic*, Parker Publishing, West Nyack, NY 1973.

Young, Frank Rudolph: *Somo-Psychic Power: Using Its Miracle Forces for a Fabulous New Life*, Parker Publishing, West Nyack, NY 1974.

Young, Frank Rudolph: *Yoga Secrets For Extraordinary Health and Long Life*, Parker Publishing, West Nyack, NY 1976.

Young, Frank Rudolph: *Zodiac Force Control: Secret of Miracle Healing and Long Life*, Parker Publishing, West Nyack, NY 1977.

Young, Frank Rudolph: *The Yogatronic Diet: Amazing New Way To A Youthful, Trim Body*, Parker Publishing, West Nyack, NY 1979.

Articles

Associated Press: 'Tantric Yoga Guru Gregorian Bivolaru Charged With Human Trafficking', *The Guardian*, 28 November 2023.

Anon.: 'The Uncertain Spy', *BBC* website, 9 February 2004 (online).

Anon.: 'Edward VIII's Links To A Mystic', *BBC* website, 6 December 2008 (online).

Anon.: 'Meet Krystal Tini of My Soul Mat in West Hollywood', *VoyageLA*, 9 September 2019 (online).

Anon.: 'New investigation for BBC Sounds and Radio 4 uncovers shocking allegations of sexual exploitation, grooming and trafficking linked to a yoga movement with followers in the UK, as British woman speaks out against accused guru Gregorian Bivolaru', *BBC* website, 9 December 2024 (online).

Anon.: 'Guido Keller', *Oblique*, n.d. (online).

Anon.: 'Michael Volin (Swami Karmananda)', *Ageless Yoga*, n.d. (online).

Anti-Defamation League: 'Active Club Network', *ADL* website, n.d. (online).

Auntie Tarot: 'Insight Institute Tarot Course', *Auntie's Tarot Blog*, 13 July 2011 (online).

Auntie Tarot: 'Insight Institute Tarot Course – Update', *Auntie's Tarot Blog*, 17 July, 2011 (online).

Auntie Tarot: 'The Insight Institute', *Auntie's Tarot Blog*, 11 September 2011 (online).

Auntie Tarot: 'A Reminiscence, Continued', *Auntie's Tarot Blog*, 13 September 2011 (online).

Auntie Tarot: 'Lind's Occult Case Book', *Auntie's Tarot Blog*, 13 October 2011 (online).

Beck, Phillipa: 'Is Yoga Cultural Appropriation?' *Full Circle Yoga*, 4 December 2019 (online).

Bernabei, Alfio: 'A Tangled Web Of Fascists, Fugitives And Secret Ops', *Searchlight*, Spring 2022.

Bhattacharya, Sanjiv: '"Call Me A Racist, But Don't Say I'm A Buddhist": Meet America's alt right', *The Observer*, 9 October 2016.

Bousfield, Jonathan: 'Gabriele D'Annunzio And The Culture of Violence', *Stray Satellite*, n.d. circa 2019 (online).

Bousfield, Jonathan: 'How Rijeka Became The World's First Fascist State', *Time Out Croatia*, n.d. circa 2019.

Burns, Kate: 'Preaching Fascism: Inside San Diego's Awaken Megachurch', *Left Coast Right Watch*, 21 February 2023 (online).

Carr, David: '*Rolling Stone* Will Replace Top Editor', *New York Times*, 29 April 2002.

Colloms, Marianne and Winding, Dick: 'Remembering The West Hampstead "Holy Man" and his Cult of Women', *Ham & High*, 23 March 2015.

Combing, Beach: 'Fiume under D'Annunzio: An Incubator of Evil', *Strange History* (online), 17 April 2014.

Cornelius: 'Dr. Alexander Cannon: A Biographical Sketch of a Friend & Acquaintance of Aleister Crowley', *Red Flame*, circa 2001 (online).

Donovan, Ned: 'The Country That Ran On Cocaine And Yoga', *Terra Nullius*, 15 April 2024 (online).

Doward, Jamie: 'Fears Mount Over Scale Of Buddhist Sect Sexual Abuse. Followers allege they were coerced into sex in 1970s and '80s with elders of UK's Triratna order', *The Guardian*, 19 February 2017.

Eliade, Mircea: 'Review Of Revolt Against The Modern World by Julius Evola', *Vremea*, Bucharest, 31 March 1935.

Evans, Christopher H.: 'Why You Should Know About The New Thought Movement', *The Conversation*, 15 February 2017 (online).

Godlee, Fiona et al.: 'Wakefield's Article Linking MMR Vaccine and Autism was Fraudulent', editorial, *British Medical Journal*, 6 January 2011 (online).

Guzmán, Gustavo: 'Miguel Serrano's Antisemitism and its Impact on the Twenty-First-Century Countercultural Rightists', *Analysis of Current Trends in Antisemitism*, Vol. 40, No. 1, January 2019.

Guerin, Cécile: 'The Yoga World Is Riddled With Anti-Vaxxers and QAnon Believers', *Wired*, 28 January 2021.

Hall, Allan: '"Ve hav vays of making you relax": How SS recommended yoga to death camp guards as a good way to de-stress', *Daily Mail*, 22 February 2012.

Hangman: 'Legacy Of Me Ne-Frego', *Noose: The Online Fascist Zine*, 5 August 2016 (online).

- Harker, Misty: 'Runic Yoga or Stadha', *Satori By M Harker* blog, n.d. circa 2013 (online).
- Hendriks, Eric C.: 'Ascetic Hedonism', *Cultural Analysis*, Vol. 11, Amsterdam 2012.
- Imy, Kate: 'Fascist Yogis: Martial Bodies and Imperial Impotence', *Journal of British Studies*, Vol. 55, No. 2, April 2016.
- Karlis, Nicole: 'Why Some New Age Influencers Believe Trump Is A "Lightworker"', *Salon*, 4 March 2021.
- Kripal, Jeffrey J.: 'Remembering Ourselves: On Some Countercultural Echoes of Contemporary Tantric Studies', *Religions of South Asia*, Vol. 1, No. 1, 28 November, 2007.
- Laddaga, Reinaldo: 'A City for Poets and Pirates', *Cabinet*, Issue 58, Summer 2015.
- Le Page, Michael: 'Lockdowns And Face Masks Really Did Help To Control Covid-19', *New Scientist*, 24 August 2023.
- Lewis, Charlie: '"There's no going back": A survivor's story of a cult's manipulation and exploitation', *Crikey*, 27 September 2024 (online).
- Locke, Christopher: 'The Yoga Tradition', *The Mystic Bourgeoisie*, 17 February 2006 (online).
- Mandrino, Marco: 'Covid Free', *Hari-Om* blog, 9 June 2021 (online).
- Mandrino, Marco: 'I Have What I Have Given (G. D'Annunzio)', *Hari-Om* blog, 3 January 2023 (onine).
- Mandrino, Marco: 'Does anyone remember, according to ancient tradition, what Yoga is for?', *Hari-Om* blog, 3 February 2023 (online).
- Mandrino, Marco: 'That Religion Called Science', *Hari-Om* blog, 31 July 2023 (online).
- Mandrino, Marco: 'R@c?sm and awareness', *Hari-Om* blog, 15 April 2024 (online).
- Mills, Ami Chen: 'Death and Taxes: When famed American yoga guru Richard Hittleman died in Santa Cruz in 1991, he left his ex-wife with a million-dollar tax bill, merciless IRS agents at the door and nowhere to turn', *Metro*, 22–29 November 1995.
- Newton, Greg Joel: 'Dr. Frank Rudolph Young and Yogametrics', *Focused Muscular Tension*, n.d. circa 2016 (online).
- O'Malley, Aidan: 'The Fascist Precursor', *Dublin Review Of Books*, May 2021.
- Pacific Antifascist Research Collective: 'People: Eric Atwood, 41, Of Manhattan Beach CA: Avowed Neo-Nazi & "Unite The Right"

Attendee', *Pacific Antifascist Research Collective* website, 28 February 2022 (online).

Rauwel, Alain: 'Henri de Lubac et le xixe siècle comme symptôme', *Archives de sciences sociales des religions*, Vol. 172, No. 4, 2015.

Rawsthorne, Sally: 'The High-Profile Sydney Yoga Studio At The Centre Of A Decidedly Un-Zen Scandal', *Sydney Morning Herald*, 26 May 2024.

Roberts, Millie: 'A Sydney Yoga Studio Compared Fully Vaxxed Freedoms To Segregation', *Junkee*, 7 October 2021 (online).

Roig-Franzia, Manuel: 'Scandal Contorts Future Of John Friend, Anusara Yoga', *Washington Post*, 28 March 2012.

Romanelli, Dave: 'Evil Yogis? The Ultimate Oxymoron', *Yes Dave*, n.d. (online).

Rosen, Richard: 'Interview with Georg Feuerstein', *Richard Rosen Yoga* (online), 10 October 1997.

Serena, Katie: '5 Fake Photos That Once Fooled Everyone But Now Fool Only Fools', *All That's Interesting*, 20 October 2017 (online).

Strelnikov: 'Gary Smith On Manoeuvres', *Who Makes The Nazis*, 27 September 2010 (online).

Strelnikov: 'Rock Against Communism: The Roots Of Sol Invictus', *Who Makes The Nazis*, 3 October 2010 (online).

Urban, Hugh B.: 'The Omnipotent Oom: Tantra and Its Impact on Modern Western Esotericism', *Esoterica: Journal of Esoteric Studies*, Vol. 3, 2001.

Valdinoci: 'A Response To Sean Ragon', *NYC Antifa*, 6 November 2014 (online).

Warzel, Charlie: 'We Sent Alex Jones' Infowars Supplements To A Lab. Here's What's In Them', *BuzzFeed News*, 9 August 2017 (online).

Waxman, Oliva B.: 'HBO's Breath Of Fire Explores The Sudden Fall Of Celebrity Yoga Teacher Guru Jagat', *Time Magazine*, 23 October 2024.

Whitman, John: 'Mussolini and the Cult of the Leader', *New Perspective*, Vol. 3, No. 3, March 1998.

Wintle, Simon: 'Insight Institute', *World Of Playing Cards*, 11 January 2013 (online).

Wood, John: 'Mike Dayton Holds Back a Hot Rod', *Oldtime Strongman*, 21 July 2016 (online).

YJ Editors: 'Recommended Yogi Reading', *Yoga Journal*, last updated 2 September 2021 (online).

Journals And Magazines

Boats and Boat Equipment, Vol. 2 No. 4, October–December 1959, Worcester Park, Surrey.
The Equinox, Vol. I, No. IV, London 1910.
The Equinox, Vol. I, No. VIII, London 1912.
The Equinox, Vol. III, No. IV, London 1939.
Fascist Quarterly, Vol. 1, London, January 1935.
Fate, Vol. 1, No. 2, Worcester Park, Surrey, December 1954.
Fate, Vol. 1, No. 3, Worcester Park, Surrey, January 1955.
International Journal: Tantrik Order Vira Sadhana, Vol. 5, No. 1, New York, Tantrik Press. Corporate author: Tantrik Order in America / International Tantrik Order, n.d. circa 1906.
Occult Review aka *London Forum*, various issues between 1908 and 1947.
Prediction, various issues between 1936 and 1996.

Dissertations

Cantú, Keith: 'Sri Sabhapati Swami and the "Translocalization" of Śivarājayoga', UC Santa Barbara 2021.
D'Orsogna, Rebecca Anne: 'Yoga in America: History, Community Formation, and Consumerism', Faculty of the Graduate School of The University of Texas at Austin 2013; published in book form under the same title by Lawchakra on 25 February 2023, ISBN-13 9781805242284.

Other Sources

Dunne, Desmond (Pseud James Lee-Richardson): *Insight School of Yoga Lessons*, Insight School of Yoga, New Malden, not dated circa 1950, mail order course.
Hari-Om blog (online).
Kasper, John, FBI Files (online).
Library of Congress Copyright Office: *Catalog of Copyright Entries. Third Series: 1953*.

Library of Congress Copyright Office: The *Catalog of Copyright Entries Third Series: 1956*.

'Magic Words' on *This American Life* hosted by Ira Glass, Chicago Public Media, radio show originally aired 15 August 2014.

Stack Exchange, 'What Biographical Information Do We Know About Author Frank Rudolph Young?' (online).

Index

n refers to a note

Above the Ruins (band)
   'No Surrender' (album) 82
   'Songs of the Wolf' (album) 82
active clubs 6
AIDS epidemic 153
Akhnaton, Pharaoh 80
Alain *Yoga for Perfect Health* 115
alcoholic drinks 102
Alexander the Great 118
alt-right 76, 79, 81, 151, 153, 158*n*7, 168*n*1
America *see* United States
American Freedom Party 5
Anderson, James *The Constitutions of the Free-Masons* 177*n*14
Anglo-American yoga 11, 109, 129
anti-semitism 52, 60
anti-vaccine movement 89, 121, 134, 155, 177*n*18, 184*n*5
Anusara yoga 3
Anusara Yoga Teacher Training Manual 3
Aphorisms of Patajañali 37
Arden, Adrienne 125, 178*n*30
   astrology column in *News of the World* 125
Armshaw, J. 100
   'Yoga and the Dowser' 172*n*10

Aryan language group speakers wrongly treated as ethnicity 26–8, 51, 64, 66–7
Asanas 32, 92, 101, 118
Ashtanga yoga 8
Atkinson, William Walker *see* Ramacharaka, Yogi
Atwood, Eric Lyle 5–6
Avalon, Arthur
   The Serpent Power 77–8
   Shakti and Shakta: Essays and Addresses on the Shâkta Tantrshâstra 77–8
Awaken Church, San Diego 136–7

Bad Guru (BBC radio programme) 154
Baker, Perry Arnold *see* Bernard, Pierre
Bannon, Steve 76–7
Bartolini, Simonetta *Yoga: Sovversivi e Rivoluzionari con D'Annunzio a Fiume* 45–6
Baruch, Bernard 144
Beach Goys (band) 6
Beck, Phillipa 70
Bennett, Allan 50
Berghaus, Günter 40
Berlusconi, Silvio 45
Bernard, Glen (father of Theos) 93–4

Bernard, Pierre 11, 14–16, 17–29, 36, 64–5, 86–7, 131
   accused of kidnapping two girls 15
   allegedly learned yoga from Silvais Hamati 18, 91–2, 93–4
   origins of 14, 19–18
   racist attitudes of 25–9
   relations with Yeats-Brown 56–8, 63
Bernard, Theos (nephew of Pierre) 87, 92–5, 109
   Hath Yoga: the Report of a Personal Experience 92, 95
   Heaven Lies Within Us 94
Besant, Annie 57
Bhagavad Gita 67–8
Bhagawan, Sri 57
Bharatiya Janata Party (BJP) 6
Bhattacharya, Sanjiv 'Call Me a Racist, But Don't Say I'm a Buddhist' 5–6, 158n7
Big Pharma 155
Bivolaru, Gregorian 154 183n1, 184n2,n3
Blavatsky, Helena 2, 32, 51, 109
Bologna Station bombing (1980) 157n1
Bose, Subhas Chandra 80
Bousfeld, Jonathan 46
Bragdon, Claude 110–1, 135
   An Introduction to Yoga 110
   Yoga for You 110–1
bodily energy centres 7
Braun, Eva 70–1
breathing 102–3, 108, 120–1
British Society of Dowsers Congress (1966) 100
British Union of Fascists 43, 47, 52, 60
British Wheel of Yoga (organisation) 69
Brunton, Paul 109, 113, 132
   'I Interview an Indian Yogi' 126
Brutal Attack (band) 82
Buddhism 50–1, 67, 112, 154
Burnett-Rae, Alan *Aleister Crowley: a Memoir of 666*: 173n12

Call-Curci, Madam 118
Callan-Thompson, Julia (mother of Stewart Home) 1–2
Cannon, Alexander 106–7, 109
Cantú, Keith 35
Carli, Mario 40
CasaPound movement 10
'Cavalcare la Tigre' (album) 82
Chamberlain, Houston Stewart 72
Charles Atlas body-building system 127–8
Choudhury, Bikram, accusations of sexual assault by 4
Christian libertarianism 9
Christianity 24, 121–2, 134, 151
Church of Satan 15
Clarkstown Country Club 16, 58, 91
Codrianu, Corneliu 73
cognitive priming 11–12
Comisso, Giovanni 40–4
   Il porto dell'amore 42–3
   Le mie stagioni 43

Index

Conspirituality (podcast) 7
Conspirituality: How New Age Conspiracy Theories Became a Health Threat (podcast) 7–8
Conway, Roger 142
Cooper, Gary 54, 59
Cosmopolitan (magazine) 62–3
Coué, Emile 23, 160n17
Covid-19 pandemic 1, 9, 121, 134, 155
 see also anti-vaccine movement
Crompton, Vera *Palmistry for Everyone* 125
Crowley, Aleister 32, 34–5, 83, 120, 126, 138, 173n12
 influence on Fuller of 48–52, 57
 Eight Lectures on Yoga 35
Crowley, Aleister and J.F.C. Fuller 'The Temple of Solomon the King IV' 50
Cult of Youth (band) 83
Current 93 (band) 'Hitler as Kalki' (album) 83

D'Annunzio, Gabriele 10, 38–46
 erection of statue in Trieste 45
D'Orsogna, Rebecca Anne 'Yoga in America: History, Community Formation and Consumerism' 25, 27–8
Dadaist movement 76
Daily Mail 66–7, 70–1, 166n11
David-Neel, Alexandra 109
Day, Harvey 104–15
 About Yoga 105–10
 Breath of Life 173n22
 Encyclopaedia of Natural Health and Healing 172n2
 The Occult Illustrated Dictionary 105–6, 172n2
 Practical Yoga for Women 63–4
 The Study of Practical Yoga 105, 108–9, 114
 You, Too, Can Write for Money 105, 109
De Michelis, Elizabeth *A History of Modern Yoga: Patanjali and Western Esotericism* 157n6
De Vries, Blanche (wife of Pierre Bernard) 16, 17
death and longevity 108, 117, 139
Death in June (band) 83
Deep Contraction (*asana*) 117–8
Deer, Brian 184n5
Delaney, Walter (pseud of Schaumberger) *Ultra-Psychonics* 99, 171n8
Desmond, Shaw 118
Devi, Indra 17, 87–8, 96–103, 132
 Forever Young, Forever Healthy 97, 98–100, 171n2
 Yoga: the Technique of Health and Happiness 97
 Yoga for Americans 100–2
 Yoga for You 100–2
Devi, Savitri 36–7, 79–83
 belief in Hitler as Kalki 80–1, 83
 The Lightning and the Sun 80–1
diet 101, 149

Dinkarswami, Pundit 'Strange
    Feats of the Yogis' 126
Disperata, La ('The Desperate'
    military company) 43
Djurdjevic, Gordan *India and the
    Occult* 34
downward dog 92
Dukes, Sir Paul Henry 16, 17, 56,
    86, 90–2
  presents BBC tv programmes
    on yoga (1948-9) 90–1
  *The Unending Quest: Auto-
    biographical Sketches* 90–1
  Yoga for the Western World 92,
    170*n*8
  *The Yoga of Health, Youth and
    Joy* 92
Duncan, Derek 42
Dunne, Desmond 35, 88, 116–28
  see also Lee-Richardson,
    James; Leigh, James

Edda (Norse mythology) 79
Eden, Richard 125–6
Egg of the Universe Yoga Studio
    155
Eisenschim, Dr. 145
El Krishnar, Maranedi *see* Young,
    Frank Randolph
Eliade, Mircea 37, 72–6
  Yoga: Immortality and Freedom
    74–6
Elliott, D.J. 20
Ellis, Albert and Roger Conway
    The Art of Erotic Seduction
    142
Equinox (journal) 49, 50
Evans, Christopher H. 8

Evans, Colin 125–6
Evans-Wentz, W.Y. 109
Everyman (magazine) 61
Evola, Julius 10, 36, 72–84, 86
  Man Against the Ruins 82
  *Revolt Against the Modern
    World* 72, 82
  *The Yoga of Power: Tantra
    Shakti and the Secret Way*
    76–9

Fascist Quarterly 52
fascist yoga 6, 35–6
  post-war development of 86–8
fascists and fascism 37
  countercultural fascism 5, 36,
    44, 81
  origins of 38
  see also fascist yoga; Italian
    fascism; Nazism
Fate (magazine) 124–5, 178*n*30
Feuerstein, Georg 69
  *The Essence of Yoga: a Contri-
    bution to the Psychohistory of
    Indian Civilization* 69
  *The Yoga Tradition: its History,
    Literature, Philosophy and
    Practice* 69
Field, Sidney 97, 171*n*2
Fiume *see* Rijeka
Flowers, Stephen 84
Folan, Lilias 88
Foucault, Michel 25
Francis, P.G. *Yoga: the Amazing
    Life Science* 115
Franco, General Francisco 60
Freemasonry 112, 119, 121,
    177*n*14

Index

Friend, John 3–4
   Anusara Yoga Teacher Training Manual 3
Friends of the Western Buddhist Order 154
Full Circle Yoga (website) 70
Fuller, J.F.C. 34, 36, 47–53, 102
   influence of Crowley on 48–52, 57
   visit to Nazi Germany by 47–8
   'Half-Hours with Famous Mahatmas' 49
   The Star in the West: a Critical Essay upon the Works of Aleister Crowley 50
   Yoga: a Study of the Mystical Philosophy of the Brahmins and Buddhists 50–1
Futurist movement 40, 76

Gabor, Eva 96
Gandhi, Mahatma 65
Garbo, Greta 96
Gardner, Martin *Fads and Fallacies in the Name of Science* 149
Gaucho (pseud of Frank Randolph Young)
Genghis Khan 80
German Faith Movement 66
Germany
   Nazi era 37, 66–71, 165n1
   Nuremberg Rally (1937) 64
   see also Nazism
Gobineau, Arthur de 72
Goebbels, Joseph 67
Goldberg, Elliott *The Path of Modern Yoga* 98, 101

Goldberg, Michelle 96
Grant, Rex (pseud of Frank Randolph Young)
'grids' 7
Griggs, Katie 4
Guénon, René 10, 73
Gune, Jagannath Ganesh 101
Guru Jagat *see* Griggs, Katie
Guyot, Felix 117, 120, 122, 138, 144
   Yoga for the West 112–3

Hackett, Paul G. 93–4
   Theos Bernard: the White Lama: Tibet, Yoga and American Religious Life 22
Haich, Elisabeth 95
Hamati, Sylvais 18–22, 86
   allegedly taught yoga to Bernard 18, 93–4
Hardy, Sam (pseud of J.F.C. Fuller)
Hari-Om Yoga School 9
Harker, Misty 83–4
Harry Ransom Center 55
Hatha yoga 23, 32
   Hatha Yoga Pradipika 51
Hathaway, Henry 59
Hauer, Jakob Wilhelm 36, 66–71, 76
   on the *Bhagavad Gita* 67–8
headstands 2, 44, 61–63, 91–2, 99–101, 123–4, 133
Hemingway, Ernest 144
Here's Health (magazine) 124, 127
Here's Health Family Guide 127
Hermetic Order of the Golden Dawn 15, 34, 119

Hettinger, Theodor 133
Himmler, Heinrich 66−8
Hindu nationalism 67, 76
Hinduism 44, 51−2, 66−7, 80, 112
   caste system 25, 27, 41, 52, 68, 80
   neo-Hindiusm 37−8, 41, 70−1, 112
Hitler, Adolf 1, 6, 25, 39, 47, 60, 64−5, 67, 70, 73, 80−1
   50th birthday parade 47−8
   Devi's belief in Hitler as Kalki 83
   Mein Kampf 72
Hittleman, Linda (wife of Richard) 129, 136, 180*n*1
Hittleman, Richard 2, 11, 88, 129−37, 180*n*1
   death of 136
   television series by 2, 129−30, 153
   Be Young with Yoga 132−3
   Guide for the Seeker 130−1, 132
   Guide to Yoga Meditation 129−30, 132
   Yoga: the 8 Steps to Health and Peace 134−5
   Yoga for Health 131
   Yoga for Physical Fitness 133−4
   Yoga, Philosophy and Meditation: an Interpretation 133−4
Hoffman, Martha 18
Hoover, Herbert 144
Hopkins, Bill 1−2, 157*n*1
Hopp, Zella 15
Hornibrook, F.A. *The Culture of the Abdomen* 114

Hoskin, Cyril Henry *see* Rampa, Lobsang T.
Houdini, Harry 14, 23
Hustler's University 151
Huxley, Julian 118

Imy, Kate 48, 54−5
   Fascist Yogis 56−7, 58−9
Insight Institute School of Personal Analysis and Development 125−6, 178*n*31
Insight School of Yoga 113, 118−20, 123, 125, 127
International Journal: Tantrick Order (IJTO) 20−1, 28
internet 153
Ionescu, Nae 73−4, 167*n*6
Iron Guard (Romanian fascist movement) 72, 73−4
isometric exercises 133
Italian fascism 36, 38−46, 73
Italian Regency of Carnaro 38, 46
   Carta del Carnaro 42
Italy
   Bologna Station bombing (1980) 157*n*1
   Years of Lead (1960-80) 1, 81

Jaquin, Noel 125
Johnson, William 5
Jones, Alex, and Infowars 116−7, 127, 156, 176*n*2
Jünger, Ernst 42−3
   Storms of Steel 42, 73

Kadetsky, Elizabeth *The Path of Modern Yoga* 97
Kali Yuga (4th world age) 79, 80

Index

Karlis, Nicole 'Why Some New Age Influencers Believe Trump is a 'Lightworker'" 167*n*15
Kasper, John 33, 161*n*3
Keller, Guido 36, 39−46, 161*n*10, 162*n*5, 163*n*16
Kelly, Gerald 59
Kemp, Minnie 175*n*1
Kent, Howard 131
Khalsa, Harbhajan Singh 4
Kripal, Jeffrey J. *Remembering Ourselves* 22
Krishnamacharya, Tirumalai 97−8
Krummer, Siegfried 84
Kundalini yoga 4, 79, 102, 134, 148
Kuvalayananda, Swami *see* Gune, Jagannath Ganesh

Laddaga, Reinaldo 43−4
Lawrence, T.E. 65
Lee-Richardson, James (aka Desmond Dunne) 125, 178*n*3
 Manual and Who's Who of Spiritualism and Psychic Research 116, 124−5
 Manual of Yoga 123, 124
 Yoga for Everyman 117−22
 Yoga Made Easy 123−4
Legat School of Russian Ballet 91
Legion of the Archangel Michael *see* Iron Guard
Legionary Movement *see* Iron Guard
Legionnaire Movement *see* Iron Guard
Leigh, James (pseud of Lee-Richardson) 116, 125
Leo, Gertrude 15
levitation 107
Lewis, Sinclair 144
Lind, Frank *My Occult Case Book* 125
Lionquest Fitness (website) 139
Lives of a Bengal Lancer, The (film) 59, 64
Locke, Christopher 69
Los Angeles Times 139
lotus position 41, 61−3
Love, Robert 14, 16, 25, 27, 93−4
 The Great Om: the Improbable Birth of Yoga in America 18−24, 59, 62−3, 94
Love and Other Drugs (film) 150
Lovinescu, Vasile 73
Lyon, Jeff 139

Magic of Chantromatics, The 171*n*8
Maharshi, Ramana 131−2
mail-order courses 116−7, 120, 126−8, 141, 143, 151, 153
 see also yoga: mail-order courses
Make America Great Again movement (MAGA) 8
Make It New bookshop 33−4
Mandrino, Marco 9−11
Mann, Thomas 118
Marby, Friedrich 84
Marinetti, F.T. 40

Marquès-Rivière, J. *Tantrik Yoga: Hindu and Tibetan* 111
Marsh, Alec *John Kasper and Ezra Pound* 33–4
masculinity cult 151
Mass Observation (MO) survey 122–3, 177*n*24
Matthesius, Jurgen 136
Maugham, W. Somerset 59
McFadden, Bernarr 106
McLaurin, Hamish 64–5
   Eastern Philosophy for Western Minds 25–7
McPherson, Aimee Semple 144–5
Mike Marvel Dynaflex muscle-building course 139–40
Mills, Ami Chen 131, 136
MMR vaccine 155, 184*n*5
modern postural practice 4, 7, 11–12, 24, 32, 35–6, 86–7, 89, 90–2, 96, 113–5, 117, 127, 134, 151, 153–6, 157*n*6
modern yoga 4, 17–18, 23, 153–4
Montalban, Madeline 125–6
   and Tarot 179*n*33
Mosley, Oswald 60
Movement for Spiritual Integration into the Absolute 154
Moynihan, Michael 5
MTV 153
Mukerji, Dan Gopal 135
Mukherji, Asit Krishna 80
Müller, Eric Albert 133
Murray's Cabaret Club 1
music, underground rock and neo-folk 5-6, 82–3
Mussolini, Benito 25, 39, 60, 73

My Soul Mat Co. 89

Nashville school bombing (1957) 33, 161*n*3
National Front 36, 82
National Socialist German Workers Party (NSDAP) 37, 47
Nazi occultism 70–1
Nazism 25, 37, 47
   neo-Nazism 5–6
   and religion 66–71
New Thought movement 8–9, 23–4, 32, 34, 121, 140, 145
New Yorker 23
New Right *see* Nouvelle Droite movement
Newcombe, Suzanne 95, 131
   Yoga in Britain: Stretching Spirituality and Educating Yogis 87, 122, 170*n*17, 177*n*24
   News of the World, astrology column by Lee-Richardson 125
Newton, Greg Joel 139
Nichols, Beverley *Cry Havoc!* 60
Norris, P.E. *see* Day, Harvey
North London Buddhist Centre 154
Nouvelle Droite movement 10
Nyack yoga centre 16, 55, 58, 90, 131

O'Malley, Aidan 'The Fascistr Precursor' 44–5
occultism 6–7, 24, 35–6, 125–6
   see also Nazi occultism
odic force 149, 174*n*

INDEX

Padfield, Peter 68
Paramahamsa, Mahatma Agamya 50
Parker (publisher) 99, 141, 143, 146, 171*n*8
Peale, Norman Vincent 9
Peterson, Eugenie *see* Devi, Indra
Plato 118
Poewe, Karla *New Religions and the Nazis* 67–8
Portas, Maximiani *see* Devi, Savitri
postural practice *see* modern postural practice
Pound, Ezra 32–4, 86
  anti-communist attitudes of 34
Prediction (magazine) 115, 116, 125–7, 178*n*31, 179*n*34,*n*39
Prentice Hall (publisher) 97, 99, 132, 133
Pythagoras 118

Qabalah 52
QAnon 1, 8, 9, 81, 89–90, 136, 156

racial nationalism 41–2, 64
Ragon, Sean 83–4
Ramacharaka, Yogi 9–10, 32–4, 108, 109
  Fourteen Lessons in Yogi Philosophy and Oriental Occultism 33, 97
  Hatha Yoga 32
Rampa, T. Lobsang *Doctor from Llasa* 173*n*22
Reichenbach, Baron von 149, 173*n*22

Reill, Dominique Kirchner *The Fiume Crisis: Life in the Wake of the Hapsburg Empire* 44–5
Rele, V.G.
  The Mysterious Kundalini 113
  Yogic Asanas 113–4
religion
  and Nazism 66–71
  and yoga 50–1, 67, 112
Remski, Matthew *Practice and All is Coming* 8
Rhine, J.B. *Extra-Sensory Perception* 112
Rice, Boyd 5
Rider (publisher) 34, 170*n*17
Rijeka 38, 43–4, 46
  exhibition of D'Annunzio's occupation 44–5
Rise Above Movement (RAM) 6
Rivière, Jean-Marie *see* Marquès-Rivière, J.
Rolling Stone (magazine) 16
Romanelli, Dave 70–1
  Evil Yogis?: the Ultimate Oxymoron 166*n*11
Romania 73–4, 154
Rosen, Richard 69
Rosenberg, Alfred *Myth of the Twentieth Century* 72–3
runic yoga 83–4
Rutherfurd, Margaret Stuyvesant (wife of Paul Dukes) 15–16, 90

Sadler, Dr. 145
Sangh, Rashtriya Swayamsevak 6
Sanhita, Shiva 52

Sanskrit 4, 64
Sarasvati, Swami Dayanand 49
Saraswati, Sivananda *Yogic Home Exercises* 109
Schaumberger, Joseph 99, 171*n*8
Secrets from Beyond the Pyramids 171*n*8
Sedgwick, Mark 73–4
Serrano, Miguel 80–1, 84
sexual abuse 3–4, 6, 8, 50, 154–5
sexual advice 65, 111, 141, 147
Shaktism 77
shoulder stands 62, 101
Sinclair, Upton 'How I Discovered Telepathy' 126
Singleton, Mark *Yoga Body* 23, 114
Sinkram courses 140
Skrewdriver (band) 82
smoking 102
Socrates 136
Sol Invictus 'Against the Modern World' (album) 82–3
Somenzi, Mino 40, 41
Spengler, Oswald 72
Spring, Clara 17
Steiger, Brad *Psychic City Chicago* 138–9
Sternhell, Zeev *The Birth of Fascist Ideology* 38
Strange History (blog) 41
Stuart, Grace *Gland Treatment for Renewal, or, Rejuvenation of the Body Through Applied New Thought* 112
Students of Western Yoga (organisation) 170*n*8
sun salutations 92, 104

Sundaram, Seetharaman *Yogic Physical Culture, or, The Secret of Happiness* 63, 165*n*25
Sunshine, Spencer *Neo-Nazi Terrorism and Countercultural Fascism* 5
Swanson, Gloria 96, 101
Sydney Yoga Studio 184*n*6,*n*7
Syman, Stefanie *The Subtle Body: the Story of Yoga in America* 22–4

Tantra (Tantrism) 77–8
Tantrik Order Journal 28
Tantrik Order of America 14–15, 20, 28
Tara Yoga Centre 154
Tarot 5, 116, 178*n*31, 179*n*33,*n*38
Tate, Andrew 151
Terza Posizione movement 10
Testa di Ferro, La (newspaper) 40
Theosophical Society 15
This American Life (radio programme) 99, 171*n*8
Thorson (publisher) 115, 170*n*17
Thorsson, Edred *see* Flowers, Stephen
Tietke, Mathias *Yoga im Nationalsozialismus: Konzepte, Kontraste, Konsequenzen* 66, 70
Tini, Krystal 89–90
Tirath, Swami Ram 20
Treaty of Rapallo (1920) 46
Tree of Life 52
Trieste, exhibition of D'Annunzio's occupation 44–5

INDEX

Triratna organisation, sexual abuse in 154–5
Trump, Donald 5, 8–9, 39, 81, 89, 167*n*15
Trungpa, Chogyam 69
Tryphonopoulos, Demetres P. 33

United States, yoga in 3, 6, 11, 24, 27–8, 62, 109, 124, 129–30
Urban, Hugh B. 22–3
  The Omnipotent Oom 18

Vanderbilt family 16
Venta, Krishna 145
Vivekananda, Swami 49
Volin, Michael 88
Vremea (newspaper) 74

Wakefield, Andrew 184*n*5
Wase, Charles *The Inner Tradition and Yoga* 111–2
Weber, Eric *How to Pick Up Girls* 142
Wertheim, Viola (wife of Theos Bernard) 92
Wertheim, Viola and Diana 28, 160*n*7
Whitaker, Alma 'Weird Occult Creeds Thrive Among Stars' 59
White, David Gordon 98
White, E.B. 23
white supremacy 6, 28–9
Whitman, Edward *Astro-Kinetics* 125
Wicca 3, 4
witchcraft 4
Wolf Age *see* Kali Yuga

Wolfe, Thomas 144
women, and self-help books 146
Woodhouse, John 40–1
Woodroffe, Sir John *see* Avalon, Arthur
Wrench, Evelyn (cousin of Yeats-Brown) *Francis Yeats-Brown: a Portrait* 55–6, 59–61, 64–5, 164*n*3

Yeats-Brown, Francis 17, 25, 26, 36, 43, 54–65, 87, 95, 107, 118, 164*n*11
  relations with Bernard 56–8, 63
  Bengal Lancer 54, 57–8, 61
  Caught by the Turks 57
  Dogs of War 60, 61
  Golden Horn 58, 61
  Lancer at Large 58, 61
  Yoga Explained 58, 61–3, 92
  Yoga for You 62–3
Yesudian, Selvarajan and Elisabeth Haich *Yoga and Health* 95
Yockey, Francis Parker *Imperium: the Philosophy of History and Politics* 83
yoga 17
  academic research in 157*n*6
  claims of Aryan origin 25–9, 79, 104, 107–8
  claims of healing powers 3, 100–1, 106, 121
  claims of Indian origin 4, 17, 35–6
  mail-order courses on 116–9, 123–4, 127–8

and religion 50–1, 67, 112
see also Anglo-American yoga; Anusara yoga; *asanas*; Ashtanga Yoga; breathing; fascist yoga; Hatha yoga; headstands; isometric exercises; Kundalini yoga; modern postural practice; modern yoga; runic yoga; sun salutations; Tantric yoga; 'yogism'
Yoga: Unione di spiriti liberi tendenti alla perfezione (journal) 40
YOGA (group) 36, 38, 40–6
Yoga Journal 75
yogametrics 113
'yogism' 117, 113, 119, 122–3
Yorke, Gerald J. 95
Young, Frank Randolph 88–9, 113, 132, 138–51, 164n3
    misogynistic attitudes of 141–3, 145–6
    sexual advice by 147
    Cyclomancy 140, 143–4, 147–8, 181n2
    Laws of Mental Domination, The 143
    Psychastra 145
    Secrets of Personal Psychic Power, The 144, 150
    Solar Diet 140, 148–9
    X-Ray Mind: a Krishnara Course 141–3, 148
    Yoga for Men Only 145–6
    Yoga Secrets for Extraordinary Health and Long Life 140, 146–7
    Yogatronic Diet, The 139, 148–50
Younghusband, Sir Francis 118

Zapp, Paul 68–9
Zohar 52, 139–40
Zwick, Edward 150

The Pluto Press Newsletter

Hello friend of Pluto!

Want to stay on top of the best radical books we publish?

Then sign up to be the first to hear about our new books, as well as special events, podcasts and videos.

You'll also get 50% off your first order with us when you sign up.

Come and join us!

Go to bit.ly/PlutoNewsletter